"This is the most comprehensive book on acne where both physical and psychological managements are most thoroughly discussed. Moreover, this book is written with amazing empathy and sensitivity for the sufferers. To call this a book on acne is a gross understatement. In all fairness, it is in fact a book on life as discussed through the topic of acne. I would like to congratulate Dr. Fried that only he, with dual expertise in dermatology and psychology and boundless compassion and mastery of life, could have written this book."

> —*John Koo, MD, professor and vice chairman in the Department of Dermatology and director of the Psoriasis Treatment Center at the University of California, San Francisco, Medical Center; boar*

"Finally: A book that gets to the heart of the psychological aspects of acne! Dr. Fried is the premiere doctor in the field of psychodermatology—and offers practical advice on not only healing the emotional triggers of this condition that robs one of self-esteem, but also treating it with the latest advances in skin care. This is a must read for anyone who's battling regular breakouts."

> —*Valerie Latona, Deputy Editor/Beauty Director,* Shape

"In *Healing Adult Acne*, Dr. Fried has successfully accomplished what so many physicians cannot, he has taken a complex subject and put it in the grasp of everyone, whether acne sufferer, therapists who work with skin disorders, or family physicians. This book is an invaluable resource for anyone interested in the many and varied types acne, their causes, and the attendant emotional trauma accompanying this disfiguration. This book will forever be my go-to source when discussing the emotional and physical causes of acne with my patients."

> —*Steven R. Howard, Ph.D., psychologist in private practice on Central Park West, New York, NY, who often treats patients suffering from the emotional trauma of skin and related disorders and member of the Association of Psycocutaneous Medicine.*

"*Healing Adult Acne* is an important new tool for our medical toolbox. The recognition and validation of the adult with acne has been a long time coming. Through a series of exercises, Dr. Fried helps acne sufferers to understand their disease and the medical and psychological impact that it has on their lives. He rationally explores proven therapy and helps to debunk common myths and expose the abundance of false claims that plague the over-the-counter acne market. He helps patients to determine when self-treatment is failing and when professional help is in order. In essence, he confirms the notion that the only real mistake in acne therapy is undertreatment and undervaluing the devastating emotional toll it takes on patients. This book will help not only patients-to-be suffering in silence, but also those already undergoing therapy who need more detailed knowledge. Education is the key to appropriate medical and psychological therapy for acne."

—*Hilary Baldwin, MD, associate professor and vice chair in the Department of Dermatology at the State University of New York at Brooklyn, acne expert and lecturer*

"This book offers an excellent explanation of the causes of acne and the current thinking on treatment. The emotional aspects of acne are also explored, making this book an invaluable asset to any patient or family member who seeks to understand the scientific and psychological effects of acne."

—*Alan Rosenbach, MD, dermatologist in private practice in Los Angeles, CA*

Healing Adult Acne

Your Guide to Clear Skin & Self-Confidence

RICHARD G. FRIED, MD, PH.D.

New Harbinger Publications, Inc.

Publisher's Note

This publication is designed to provide accurate and authoritative information in regard to the subject matter covered. It is sold with the understanding that the publisher is not engaged in rendering psychological, financial, legal, or other professional services. If expert assistance or counseling is needed, the services of a competent professional should be sought.

Distributed in Canada by Raincoast Books

Copyright © 2005 by Richard Fried
New Harbinger Publications, Inc.
5674 Shattuck Avenue
Oakland, CA 94609

Cover design by Amy Shoup; Cover image: Ryan McVay/Getty Images; Acquired by Melissa Kirk; Edited by Jessica Beebe; Text design by Tracy Marie Carlson

Library of Congress Cataloging-in-Publication Data

Fried, Richard G.
  Healing adult acne : your guide to clear skin and self-confidence / Richard G. Fried.
    p. cm.
  ISBN 1-57224-415-1 (pbk.)
  1. Acne. 2. Acne—Treatment. I. Title.
  RL131.F75 2005
  616.5'3—dc22
                          2005018914

New Harbinger Publications' Web site address: www.newharbinger.com

07   06   05

10   9   8   7   6   5   4   3   2   1

First printing

This book is dedicated to the people who taught me about life and to those who gave me the privilege of learning about and touching theirs: my family, friends, and patients.

Contents

Acknowledgments

In order to be a healer, one must understand the human condition and believe in the goodness and power of the human spirit. In order to heal, one must believe that healing is possible. I believe with certainty that the majority of people are fundamentally good and, if given the chance, will choose to find happiness and do the right thing. With belief, support, and encouragement, the human organism can heal and flourish. I believe that all of us have the innate capacity to heal the wounds of the skin and the soul. With healing comes strength and knowledge, not fragility. The journey through life is punctuated by many opportunities, successes, and failures. Each of these experiences provides us an opportunity for growth and happiness.

I have been blessed with many mentors throughout my personal and professional life. My parents and brother taught me the power of love, strength, and emotional healing. My wife has enriched my world with her endless integrity, love, beauty, strength, perseverance, and support. My wonderful children touch my soul, and their innate goodness gives a deeper meaning to my life.

There are many dermatologists who have been gracious enough to share with me their knowledge and kindness. The following list is by no means complete, and I sincerely apologize in advance to anyone inadvertently omitted. I extend my sincere thanks to Alan Shalita, MD; Ed Heilman, MD; Neil Brody, MD, Ph.D.; Yelva Lynfield, MD; Hilary Baldwin, MD; Caroline Koblenzer, MD; Peter Koblenzer, MD; Steven Feldman, MD, Ph.D.; Guy Webster, MD, Ph.D.; John Koo, MD; Larry Eichenfield, MD; Aditya Gupta, MD, Ph.D.; Mark Lebwohl, MD; Alice Gottlieb, MD, Ph.D.; Jim Marks, MD; Diane Thiboutot, MD; Diane Berson, MD; and Jeff Miller, MD.

I wish to thank Melissa Kirk at New Harbinger Publications for her vision realizing the importance of a book on acne and her invaluable organizational direction. I also sincerely thank copyeditor Jessica Beebe for her excellent input and direction. I applaud New Harbinger Publications for their commitment to excellence and meticulous attention to detail and documentation of all facts presented in the book.

Introduction

Living with acne can be a nightmare. How do I know this? Because people like you have educated me. Initially as a Ph.D.-level clinical psychologist and later as an MD board certified dermatologist, I've had the privilege of listening to many people and learning about the devastating effects that acne can produce. It has become clear to me that skin and emotion are intimately and intricately linked. Acne can be responsible for stress, depression, anxiety, self-consciousness, social withdrawal, job impairment, and intimacy difficulties. Conversely, these and other negative emotions can also cause the onset or worsening of acne. This is a cruel double whammy: your acne gets worse, you feel terrible and stressed, and as a result your acne worsens. What kind of nasty joke is that?

I am a doctor who truly understands the two-way street linking acne and emotion. This book is intended to be not only a source of accurate information but also an invaluable guide for better living. It is for anyone who has or has had acne. Why? Because if you currently suffer with acne or have suffered with it in the past, you may carry emotional baggage that can worsen your acne and self-image and compromise your ability to lead a happy life. Since almost everyone either presently suffers from acne or has suffered its effects in the past, this book is written for anyone who has skin.

I want you to have a clear complexion. I want you to be happy. I will share with you the truth about why acne happens and what treatments really work. I will examine the newest treatments, such as lasers, intense pulse lights, photodynamic therapy, and new medications. Skincare products like cleansers, spot gels, clearing gels, alpha hydroxy acids (AHAs), beta hydroxy acids (BHAs), botanicals, and moisturizers will be discussed. This book will examine the lies about what causes and cures acne and expose the liars who promise miraculous overnight cures. It will explore the role of stress in causing or worsening acne and, more importantly, suggest steps you can take to minimize the effects of stress on your skin, body, and psyche. I will help you identify your areas of stress that can serve as triggers for your acne.

Chapter 1 will examine the structure and function of the skin and expose the true causes of acne. In chapter 2, I'll discuss basic skin care to prevent and improve your acne. Chapter 3 will help you identify your acne triggers so that you may be able to modify your behaviors and minimize breakouts. In chapters 4 and 5, I'll review the available and emerging skin therapies and discuss how to choose the treatment options that are right for you. Chapters 6 and 7 will explore the psychological effects of acne and help you assess how acne may have affected your psyche. Chapter 8 will offer specific techniques to help you effectively deal with stress, anxiety, and depression. In chapter 9, I'll offer suggestions and exercises to enhance your social life. Chapter 10 will help you achieve the goal of living well with acne and having a full and meaningful life. The book will conclude by providing an overall perspective on acne and life.

The knowledge and skills you'll learn in this book will help you better manage your acne, your emotions, and your life. You will learn and hopefully practice simple and effective techniques to modify your perceptions and stress responses in positive ways. These techniques can improve the quality of your life and help you look and feel better. I'll provide exercises and strategies to enhance your comfort and effectiveness in social and professional situations. Thus, the goal of this book is certainly to help you have better skin, but perhaps more importantly to help you live comfortably inside it.

I

Why Me, Why Now? The Causes and Effects of Acne

Without question, you are bombarded with an overwhelming amount of confusing and incorrect information about what causes acne and which treatments work. This chapter is intended as a source of factual information to help you understand the reasons your skin breaks out and the potential physical and emotional effects of those breakouts. I believe that if you start with the real facts, the choices become easier. Before I get down to business and tell the real acne story, I would like to introduce you to Susan.

■ Susan

Rather suddenly, the seemingly endless collection of zit jokes that had amused Susan and her coworkers were no longer were funny. Since becoming the head of a division of an over-the-counter acne product company, Susan had become immersed in acne products, promotional strategies, and acne humor. Dismissive comments about the horror of a zit before the prom, troubling PMS pimples, postacne "pizza face," obviously sex-starved acne sufferers, and so forth all now sounded so insensitive.

As Susan stared into the bathroom mirror, the angry, painful, swollen cysts on her chin, cheeks, and forehead distorted her face to near grotesque proportions. Three months to the day after accepting her new position, Susan suddenly began breaking out. At age thirty-four and after an adolescence marred by only mild acne, Susan had until now taken pride in her nearly flawless complexion. The acne problems that so many of her friends experienced in their teens and twenties passed her by, and at times she pitied her friends for their bad luck and obvious lack of sophistication with regard to skin care. Susan had always washed with a gentle exfoliating cleanser followed by an oil-free moisturizer. Every skincare product she purchased was labeled *noncomedogenic* (the fancy name for products tested and found to not promote acne). She'd always removed her makeup before bed and drank at least four eight-ounce glasses of water per day. Despite the stress of her new job, she ate well, exercised regularly, avoided caffeine, drank herbal tea, and had regular facials.

How could this be happening to her, she wondered?

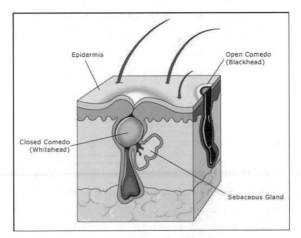

Figure 1.1   Acne Lesion: Up Close and Personal

Was this some cruel retribution for her previous insensitivity or some other moral imperfection? Had her hormones suddenly gone awry? Tears began to well in her eyes and she felt helpless, overwhelmed, and embarrassed. Where could she hide? What could she do?

ACNE FACTS

Susan is typical of the patients who fill my office. Some, like Susan, are struggling with acne for the first time. Others as teenagers had acne that subsided and returned, while many never outgrew their acne and continue to struggle with it into adulthood.

The demographics of acne are changing. Recent studies suggest that adult acne is becoming increasingly common (Goulden, Stables, and Cunliffe 1999). I can no longer reassure teenagers that they will outgrow their acne during their teen years. In fact, many will have their acne worsen substantially as they enter their twenties with more extensive and inflamed lesions. Nor can I assure young adults with pristine skin that their adult years will be free of acne miseries. Dermatologists are seeing an epidemic of acne beginning in or persisting into adulthood. Many dermatology practices actually treat more adult acne patients than teenagers. Patients cannot even be assured that their acne will cease after menopause. The exact reasons for the increase in adult acne are unclear, but many solid theories exist and will be explored in this book. One fact that is absolutely certain is that the concept of acne as a more chronic condition is changing how dermatologists view and treat the disease.

Acne vulgaris is the distasteful technical name for this ubiquitous affliction. It is composed of a variety of skin lesions: somewhere on the skin, there are some blackheads and/or whiteheads. Red bumps may or may not be present at any given time.

At least 80 percent of people experience acne at some point in their lives, and it is the most common skin disease in the United States (Plewig and Kligman 2000). Acne affects 40 to 50 million Americans (American Academy of Dermatology 2005). Despite the promises made by marketers of over-the-counter acne products and the $282 million spent on these products last year alone (Information

Resources 2004), a significant number of adult acne sufferers do not see improvement with over-the-counter products. Clearly, the available nonprescription products are inadequate to treat many acne sufferers.

Further, many myths exist about why people are afflicted with acne, and these myths have the potential to cause psychological harm. Some of these misconceptions focus on the personal hygiene and moral integrity of the acne sufferer. Such attributions can certainly challenge and diminish the perceived character of the affected person. Other theories implicate diet, allergy, cosmetics, stress, and hormones. In this chapter, I'll explain what we do know about the causes of acne.

The Physiology of Acne

In order to help you understand the true causes of your acne, I want to share with you some important facts about your skin. Understanding how your skin works and what really causes acne will enhance your ability to choose effective and legitimate treatments. This knowledge will also help you avoid bogus and ineffective approaches.

DO YOU SPEAK ZITTONESE?

Let me explain some acne terminology. There are two languages for acne, the colloquial and the medical. Of course the medical has the big, long, fancy-sounding names. Actually, there is a purpose for the "medicalese." It is a universally accepted norm of descriptions shared by medical professionals that allows for precision of description. In this way, health-care professionals can communicate precisely and be assured that what is being described is clear and understandable. This permits accurate descriptions, correct diagnoses, and appropriate treatment plans.

Colloquially, we call acne lesions zits, pimples, and blemishes. Medically, we call them *comedones* (blackheads and whiteheads), *papules* (raised red bumps), *pustules* (raised white bumps), *cysts* (firm rubberlike balls beneath the skin), and *nodules* (deep, often tender, large rubberlike balls beneath the skin). The openings in the skin that all acne lesions arise from are colloquially called pores and medically called *hair follicles*. Throughout the book, these two terms will be used interchangeably.

IT'S ALL ABOUT THE PORES

Pores are the tiny openings in your skin that are present everywhere on the body except the palms and soles. Pores, or hair follicles, extend from the top layer of the skin (the *epidermis*) all the way down to the fat. There are specialized oil-producing glands called *sebaceous glands* attached to each hair follicle (see figure 1.1). If you are genetically destined to have large, very productive sebaceous glands, you have oily skin. In contrast, people with small, minimally productive sebaceous glands tend to have dry skin. In women, most of the pores on the face, chest, and back have tiny, light hairs coming out of them called *vellus hairs*. These vellus hairs are largely invisible to the naked eye. Therefore, while hair density in women varies by genetics, most have less of the dense and dark facial hair seen in men, whose follicles are more often filled with thick, darker hairs called *terminal hairs*.

Normal pores. Specialized cells called *keratinocytes* line all of the pores, or hair follicles, on your skin. These hair follicle lining cells live for only a finite period of time, then they die. These dead cells slough off; that is, they are shed or cast off and are replaced by new, healthy cells. The keratinocytes are microscopic, so they are invisibly shed. A few are lost to the washcloth or the stream of water in the shower, while others are lost to an astringent pad or the brush of a fingertip. This replacement of lining cells is an ongoing renewal process that occurs throughout your life.

Acne-prone pores. In contrast to normal pores, acne-prone pores are those with lining cells that become abnormally sticky. These sticky keratinocytes can no longer be shed one at a time, but instead become clumps that clog the hair follicle. This clogged pore is the basis of every pimple in every individual, regardless of age, ethnicity, or race. The clogged follicle appears on the skin as either a blackhead or whitehead. If the sticky keratinocytes remain sealed within the pore and are not exposed to oxygen, a whitehead is formed. In contrast, if these keratinocytes are exposed to oxygen, they become oxidized, and a blackhead results. A bacterium called *Propionibacterium acnes* (*P. acnes*) is often trapped in the acne-prone pore. This bacterium thrives in the clogged pore and is fed by the oil produced by the sebaceous gland.

Whether you are sixteen, thirty-five, sixty-one, or ninety-six years old, the bottom-line story is the same: If you have acne, your keratinocytes are misbehaving. Your acne lesion begins its annoying life as a microscopic clogged hair follicle, invisible to the naked eye, technically called a *microcomedone* (remember that comedones are whiteheads or blackheads). The microcomedone forms because the cells that line the follicle become abnormally thick and sticky, clogging the pore.

Specifically, your keratinocytes become abnormally thick and sticky in response to adult hormones, leading to what we colloquially call a pimple. So, the truth is that acne is really all about hair follicles and hormones. Contrary to popular myths and misconceptions, breakouts are rarely the result of poor hygiene, poor diet, or evil thoughts. They happen because you inherited a genetic predisposition that directs your keratinocytes to behave abnormally in response to adult hormones (which become active at puberty). While there are sometimes abnormal hormone levels, most acne sufferers have normal hormone levels.

Clinically, blackheads appear as black dots within an open pore. Whiteheads are small, white raised bumps. Blackheads and whiteheads usually are not inflamed. Inflamed, red-bump acne occurs in response to bacteria such as *P. acnes* trapped in the clogged pore.

The Genetics of Acne

Acne runs in families, but in an unpredictable way. Children of acne sufferers are definitely more likely to suffer from acne than children of parents who did not have acne. However, many children whose parents suffered terrible acne don't ever develop acne, while some children of people with flawless skin go on to develop severe acne. Even identical twins can differ in the amount of acne they experience. Therefore, it's impossible to pinpoint which parent or distant relative gave you the propensity to develop acne. You can think in terms of probability: if stubborn acne runs in the family, you should watch for the development of acne and seek prompt medical treatment.

Genetics also probably determines when your acne will begin and end. This timetable is in all likelihood somewhat modified by environmental factors such as diet, medications, stress, cosmetic use, and hygiene. For some, acne begins at puberty, while for others, the onset can be much later. Adult acne usually abates in the thirties or forties, but persistence into later decades is sometimes seen.

Hormonal Factors

Almost all acne is hormonal. There are hundreds of hormones in your body that control and modify all the organ systems, including the skin, hair, nails, heart, and brain. In short, hormones control the way you look, feel, think, and function. A specific group of hormones called *androgens* is believed to be responsible for acne. *Testosterone, androstenedione, dehydroepiandrosterone, progesterone, androsterone,* and *dihydrotestosterone*—all types of androgens—have each been implicated as active players affecting the development and worsening of acne. *Androgen* is a general term for any natural or synthetic compound that stimulates or controls the development and maintenance of masculine characteristics. Androgens are made in the testes in the male, in the ovaries in the female, and in the adrenal glands in both sexes. Both men and women have androgens circulating in the body, with levels generally being much higher in men. So it is predominantly the male hormones that are perpetrating all this misery.

People rarely get pimples before puberty because the testes and ovaries do not produce adult androgens until that time. Once androgen production begins, these hormones stimulate the keratinocytes to misbehave (become abnormally thick and sticky) in predisposed people. Again, acne develops because the hair follicle lining cells respond abnormally to these androgens, usually not because of abnormal androgen levels. Most acne lesions are an abnormal response to normal or, at most, minimally abnormal hormones. Thus, to reiterate, the majority of pimples result from pore lining cells overreacting to normal androgens.

A small percentage of acne occurs because of abnormally elevated androgens. When androgens are elevated, it is important that they be addressed, since in addition to causing acne, they can also be associated with infertility, heart disease, and diabetes. Clues suggesting possible hormonal excess include

- acne that is extremely resistant to treatment,

- excessive facial and body hair,

- hair loss,

- irregular periods,

- midcycle breakthrough bleeding,

- breast tenderness or discharge,

- deepening of the voice,

- enlargement of the clitoris, and

- abdominal pain or enlargement.

Having one or some of these signs does not necessarily mean that your levels are abnormal. However, if any are present, I suggest that you consult a dermatologist or your primary care physician. Your doctor will do a thorough physical examination and review your medical history to determine whether laboratory or imaging studies are necessary. If there is suspicion of hormonal excess, testing for exact levels of some adrenal and ovarian hormones (such as androstenedione, dehydroepiandrosterone, progesterone, androsterone, dihydrotestosterone, and free and total testosterone) may be requested. Levels of the pituitary hormone *prolactin* and a circulating protein, *sex hormone binding globulin,* may be tested as well.

Since true hormonal problems are rare, let's return to the stubborn, miserable acne that plagues people with normal hormone levels. Subtle and modest elevation of androgens or overresponsiveness of the hair follicles probably accounts for most of your breakouts. These small changes are usually undetectable with standard blood tests. We know that androgens can be slightly elevated by many factors, including stress (which directly increases production of androgens by the testes, ovaries, and adrenal glands), oral supplementation with androgens such as those found in bodybuilding formulations, medical conditions leading to excess production by the ovaries or adrenal glands, and possibly from hormone supplementation in foods we ingest (such as bovine growth hormone in milk). The reasons the pore lining cells overreact to these subtle changes are less clear. Current research efforts are focusing on the cascade of events leading to these abnormal cellular responses. These studies will undoubtedly yield more effective interventions for the control of acne.

The Role of Stress

Stress is defined as any occurrence that disrupts the psychological and physiological well-being of an organism. There are physical stressors such as pain, hunger, heat, cold, restraint, excessive exertion, and exhaustion. While emotional or psychological stress is considerably harder to define, I believe that you will agree that relationship difficulties, loss of a loved one, job hassles, and financial troubles seem like obvious stressors. It is sometimes hard to define and pinpoint exactly which of the many demands and looming possibilities in your life stress you the most.

Regardless of the origin of the stress, a wide body of research confirms that stress has deleterious effects on many organ systems, the skin included. Stress can act to cause acne by several mechanisms. It can affect the ovaries, testes, and adrenal glands, leading to release of androgens throughout the body; it can cause direct hormonal changes at the level of the hair follicle; and it can increase the release of inflammatory chemicals, leading to more inflamed acne. Stress can interfere with sleep, encourage poor eating habits, disrupt exercise routines, increase fatigue, and decrease adherence to good skincare regimens. A 2003 study published in the *Archives of Dermatology* (Chiu and Kimball) confirmed that stress can cause changes in the hair follicle that directly contribute to the formation of acne lesions. Zouboulis and Bohm (2004) demonstrated a direct effect of stress on the hormones within the hair follicle. The contribution of stress to any given acne breakout is unknown. However, the benefits of stress management techniques for overall health and quality of life are extremely important. In chapter 8, I'll discuss ways you can learn to better manage your stress.

TYPES OF ACNE

In general, dermatologists first describe acne as being either *noninflammatory* (blackhead and whitehead) or *inflammatory* (red and tender bump) acne. Acne in women is sometimes further classified according to its association with time of month (premenstrual) and time of life (menopausal). Other factors can also influence acne. Infertility treatments and many medications can cause or worsen acne. Subtypes such as pyoderma faciale and acne fulminans are rare but very serious forms of acne requiring prompt and aggressive treatment. Acne rosacea is also relatively uncommon, but it requires specialized treatment. In this section, I'll discuss each of these types of acne and its causes.

Why Adult Acne?

Adult acne occurs for the same basic reasons as adolescent acne. The follicular lining cells respond abnormally to androgens, and there is often inflammation. What remains unclear is why we are seeing an epidemic of adult acne. Some experts think that adult acne may be caused by subtle hormonal changes that do not appear on standard blood tests, others blame alterations in the responsiveness of the hair follicle, while still others focus on diet and hormone and antibiotic supplementation of our food sources, and finally many suggest that modern life stresses are contributors.

Adult acne lesions tend to be deeper, more cystic (feeling like a rubber ball), and more localized to the center of the face and the jawline than adolescent acne. The skin of an adult is sometimes less tolerant of acne than an adolescent's and will form scars. It is not unusual to see patients who describe a history of excellent skin that is now becoming marred by new scars from acne. Janice, a thirty-nine-year-old stay-at-home mother summed up succinctly the frustration of adult acne: "Zits and wrinkles at the same time! This is just not fair!"

Inflammatory Acne

Now, the plot thickens. Why is it that you don't simply develop blackheads and whiteheads, or noninflammatory acne? What causes inflammatory acne—the red, raised bumps or the deep, tender lumps that form beneath the skin? The answer is that there is a cascade of events triggered by the same relatively innocuous bacteria trapped within the clogged pore (follicle) that causes noninflammatory acne. These events are exacerbated when your immune system overreacts.

BACTERIA AND INFLAMMATORY ACNE

The bacterium that causes most acne, *P. acnes*, is not generally implicated in serious skin infections. However, in the setting of inflammatory acne, *P. acnes* releases and recruits a host of chemicals that can cause a great deal of inflammation and damage in the skin. *P. acnes* is a resilient and highly adaptive bacterium that grows on virtually anything and can repair itself when damaged. It thrives in an environment that is dark, relatively oxygen free, and rich in fat. This precisely describes the environment within a clogged hair follicle. *P. acnes* flourishes within clogged pores, and as a result, its by-products cause substantial irritation within and around the follicle. Sometimes, the follicle can even rupture. This releases the contents of the pore into the skin and can elicit a tremendous amount of inflammation. This inflammation accounts for the red and tender lesions of inflammatory acne.

IMMUNE SYSTEM OVERREACTIVITY

You have just learned how *P. acnes* contributes to the red, tender bumps of inflammatory acne. However, it is also important to understand that the immune system plays a substantial role in causing and worsening inflammatory acne. Simply stated, inflammatory acne is caused in part by an overzealous response of the immune system. These red, tender acne lesions occur because your immune system, in some respects, works too well. There is a great deal of societal attention placed on enhancing immune function. We are fearful of infection and cancer and are always seeking methods to fortify ourselves. Many of us swallow vitamins and other health-promoting elixirs in the hope that we will be well prepared for a bacterial, viral, fungal, or carcinogenic attack.

There is, however, a flip side to this high degree of immune readiness and vigilance. A state of optimized readiness can result in exaggerated immune reactions to relatively benign occurrences. *P.*

acnes is a relatively wimpy bacterium. There are no cases of serious tissue or blood infection with these bacteria. But unfortunately, in many people, the immune system reacts to the presence of *P. acnes* in the hair follicles as if it were a virulent, potentially life-threatening infection. The immune system tries desperately to wall off the infected follicle by laying down fibrous scar tissue around the infection. This is exactly what can happen in response to an inflamed follicle. The end result is the formation of scar tissue that creates a downward pull on the follicle, manifesting as a sunken scar.

Effective treatments for inflammatory acne must address this excessive and potentially destructive immune response. Since stress contributes to excessive immune response, the stress management and lifestyle improvement exercises in chapters 8, 9, and 10 will help improve your acne.

Hormonal Havoc: Women and Acne

Adult acne is much more common in women than in men. This is probably related to the many hormonal changes that women must face throughout their lives. Men have only one substantial change in their hormonal status, and that occurs with increased testicular production of androgens at puberty. Thereafter, levels of self-produced androgens remain relatively constant in men through age thirty, except for modest changes in response to stress and the other factors discussed earlier. As men age, there is a gradual decrease in testosterone levels. While this may affect energy levels and libido, it rarely causes or worsens acne.

In contrast, let's look at the hormonal roller-coaster ride women face. As in men, there is an increase in androgen production at the time of puberty. Not long after relatively stable hormone levels are achieved, some women choose to take birth control pills for a variety of reasons, including regulation of menstrual periods, reduction in menstrual discomfort, acne control, and contraception. The follicles adjust to these new hormone levels, only to be challenged again by discontinuation of the oral contraceptive. Sometimes discontinuation is due to failure to renew prescriptions, lack of need for contraception, or desire to become pregnant.

A series of hormonal changes are initiated by pregnancy. If conception occurs easily, massive hormonal changes take place to maintain the pregnancy. If a woman needs medical assistance to become pregnant, fertility drugs are often used, and they create hormonal havoc. Finally, the follicles adjust to the pregnant state, only to undergo an abrupt change after delivery of the baby. Now, in the postpartum period, hormones gradually return to a relatively steady state, although intermediate levels of hormones are required to sustain milk production in women who are breastfeeding. Eventually, contraception again becomes an issue, and many women choose to return to the birth control pill. This pill, pregnancy, postpartum, pill cycle repeats itself with each subsequent pregnancy. Enough, you say? Yes, absolutely—but there's more.

Now, menopause approaches. Slowly, and unfortunately sometimes erratically, the ovaries decrease production of estrogen, resulting in more available testosterone to wreak havoc with the follicles. Some women find themselves episodically on and off hormone replacement therapy to improve quality of life and improve acne.

Given the seemingly endless hormone fluctuations throughout a woman's life, it seems inevitable that adult acne should occur. Let's take a closer look at how acne is affected by the menstrual cycle, infertility treatments, and menopause.

PREMENSTRUAL ACNE

Women have told dermatologists for many years that acne often emerges or worsens during the premenstrual period. It is only within the past two years that studies have confirmed what women already knew (Harper and Thiboutot 2003). The decrease in estrogen that occurs before the onset of the menstrual flow allows testosterone to predominate and stimulate the follicles to form acne. The severity of this common premenstrual acne flare determines the type of treatment required. Deep and very inflamed cystic lesions usually require oral medications, injections into the lesions, or both in order to avoid scarring.

INFERTILITY TREATMENT ACNE

New onset acne or worsening of existing acne is common among women undergoing treatments for infertility. Many of the agents used to induce ovulation (release of an egg by the ovary) produce hormonal changes that can wreak havoc with the skin. Inflammatory red-bump acne and deeper cystic lesions are common. Treatment options for this acne are limited, since medications that can pose even theoretical harm to the developing fetus are avoided. The scientific reality and available data suggest that any minimal absorption of *topical* (externally applied) agents through the skin is probably incapable of affecting the fetus. However, on the emotional side, no pregnant woman needs to be burdened with concern that she has done anything that could possibly harm her child. Therefore, topical retinoids (e.g., Retin-A) are avoided and only topical antibiotics such as erythromycin are recommended. Alpha and beta hydroxy acid products are believed to be safe. In extreme cases where scarring is imminent or has already occurred, treatment with oral erythromycin can be effective. This antibiotic has been shown to be safe from conception through delivery and beyond. The only consolation regarding acne caused by infertility treatment is the fact that it is usually transient, resolving after infertility treatments have been stopped.

MENOPAUSAL ACNE

Menopause is the medical name for the time in life when ovarian function dramatically declines (estrogen and testosterone production decrease) and the ovaries no longer release eggs. The absence of eggs for fertilization and diminished hormone production usually make pregnancy impossible, unless donor eggs and hormonal supplementation are used.

Menopause brings with it a host of potential challenges. While much is written about negative aspects such as hot flashes, mood changes, loss of skin elasticity, and vaginal dryness, acne is rarely discussed. The fact is that acne can and does frequently occur during the process of menopause. The exact reasons are unclear, but the relative lack of estrogen to mitigate the pro-acne effects of circulating androgens is probably a significant contributor. The good news is that menopausal acne responds well to conventional acne treatments and can usually be brought under good control. Further, most women find that menopausal acne tends to improve as the body adjusts to the new hormonal milieu that stabilizes after menopause.

Psychologically, menopausal acne can be distressing. Menopause is often a time of introspection and reflection. Some find the loss of reproductive function and the possibility of changes in attractiveness and sexual function to be emotionally difficult. The appearance of acne during this transition period can only add to the psychological burden.

The good news is underreported by our gloom-and-doom media. Many women find menopause to be an enormously liberating transition. Fears of unwanted pregnancy and the discomfort and intrusiveness of the monthly menses are no longer present. As with other transition periods in life, new freedoms and increased self-acceptance and self-confidence often emerge.

Less Common Types of Acne

Now that I've discussed the more common types and causes of acne, let's take a look at some of the less common types: pyoderma faciale, acne fulminans, and acne rosacea.

PYODERMA FACIALE AND ACNE FULMINANS

Both *pyoderma faciale* and *acne fulminans* are rare forms of extremely inflammatory acne. With pyoderma faciale and acne fulminans, red, tender, painful, and even bleeding acne lesions make a sudden appearance. It is almost as though you go to sleep without acne and wake up the next morning with severe acne. The acne sometimes literally appears overnight. Pyoderma faciale usually occurs in females, while acne fulminans usually occurs in males. The cause of these conditions is not fully understood, but both are considered severe inflammatory reactions, extreme examples of the immune system overreactivity discussed earlier in this chapter.

Pyoderma faciale and acne fulminans are more than skin-deep. Besides the extremely painful skin lesions, symptoms such as joint pains, muscle pains, and excessive fatigue are often present as well. Evidence that both these conditions are true full-body reactions is found when medical tests are performed. Abnormalities in blood tests are sometimes found, and in rare instances, there are even abnormal X-ray studies showing inflammation in the bones and joints.

Pyoderma faciale and acne fulminans are true dermatologic emergencies. If these intense forms of acne are not aggressively treated, the massive inflammation can result in extensive scarring of the skin. You can think of the underlying problem as a raging internal fire of inflammation directed against the hair follicles. Oral steroids such as prednisone (Deltasone) or methylprednisone (Medrol) are usually necessary to put out these inflammatory flames before substantial damage to the skin occurs. However, despite their wonderful anti-inflammatory effects, the steroids alone are not enough. Isotretinoin (Accutane, Sotret, Amnesteem, Claravis) is also necessary. Isotretinoin works in two ways: it corrects the underlying hair follicle abnormalities, and it also has anti-inflammatory prop-erties. The isotretinoin and steroids work in an additive fashion to clear and fix the problem.

It is extremely unlikely that you will ever develop pyoderma faciale or acne fulminans. I present them not just to convince you that there are genuine dermatologic emergencies other than a zit before the prom. My goal is to make you aware that there are times when very prompt medical attention is essential. If you think that you may have either of these conditions, call your dermatologist or primary care physician today.

ACNE ROSACEA

Determining whether you have acne vulgaris or acne rosacea is not always that easy. In contrast to acne vulgaris (which involves blackheads, whiteheads, and often red bumps), *acne rosacea* is a chronic inflammatory skin disorder characterized by persistent redness and dilated small blood vessels called *telangiectases*. Swelling, inflam-matory acnelike bumps, and a tendency toward blushing and flushing may be present. While an exhaustive discussion of acne rosacea is beyond the scope of this book, I would be remiss if I did not mention this disorder. Acne rosacea can occur together with acne vulgaris, and excluding one or the other with absolute certainty is often impossible.

Why is it important to make the distinction? Accurate diagnosis is very important because these conditions often require different treatment regimens. Common to the treatment of both acne vulgaris and acne rosacea is the use of topical and oral antibiotics. Rosacea often responds well to topical metronidazole products (Metrogel, Noritate) and, like acne vulgaris, can be improved with topical sodium sulfacetamide products (Klaron, Rosanil, Rosac, and Clenia). Acne rosacea varies tremendously in its severity. Some people with rosacea have little more than sensitive skin with mild redness. Others can have extremely exuberant redness with deep-seated and disfiguring acne nodules. Permanent swelling of the skin with enlargement of the nose, cheeks, and chin can also occur. More severe cases sometimes require laser treatments in combination with topical and oral antibiotics. Isotretinoin can be helpful in severe cases or those that don't respond to other treatments.

The bottom line here is that evaluation and accurate diagnosis, preferably by a dermatologist, will provide the best opportunity for optimal management of your skin. There are many good information resources for the diagnosis and treatment of rosacea, such as the National Rosacea Society and the American Academy of Dermatology.

AFTER THE BREAKOUT: ACNE'S TELLTALE FOOTPRINTS

As if the pimple itself is not annoying enough, there are often marks left behind at the places where the pimples were. These marks range from pink-red spots or brown spots to scars of all types. While the physical marks on the skin are visible, the emotional effects on the psyche are only felt. In this section, we'll look at the physical and emotional effects of acne.

Hyperpigmentation

Most acne sufferers are aware that red or brown spots can persist long after the active, raised, tender pimple itself goes away. These "reminder spots" are the result of the intense inflammation that surrounded the hair follicle and caused deposition of pigment into the skin. The technical name for these spots is *postinflammatory hyperpigmentation*. The spots tend to be darker and more persistent in people who have darker skin: Asians, Native Americans, and African-Americans. These spots can be very conspicuous and cause a great deal of self-consciousness. Many treatments are available to fade these marks, and they will be discussed in chapter 4.

While we tend to focus on the acne lesions, it is important for health-care providers to recognize that self-consciousness, depression, and anxiety are common emotional reactions to the hyperpigmentation. These negative emotional responses can sometimes be more troubling to you than your responses to the active acne lesions. Just when you think you are out of the woods and home free, the hyperpigmentation presents a whole new issue to deal with.

Scars

Layton and colleagues (1994) estimate that some degree of skin scarring occurs in 95 percent of acne sufferers, and the longer the acne lesions persist, the more likely scarring will occur. Scarring from acne occurs when scar tissue replaces normal skin and skin structures. Scarring is the end result of tissue destruction. The tissue destruction accompanying acne is usually caused by vigorous inflammation resulting from both the local effects of *P. acnes* and its by-products and immune system overreactivity to this relatively benign bacterium. Many factors can influence the extent of scarring and type of scar produced. Genetics plays some role, because some people have skin that scars more easily than others regardless of age, color, or ethnicity. However, as a general rule, fair-skinned people tend to scar more easily, while darker-skinned people tend to have more problems with pigmentation. Long-standing acne lesions and those that have been picked at are more likely to scar.

Emotional Effects

Describing and measuring the physical scars from acne is very straightforward. We use terms such as ice pick scarring (sharp indentations) and *atrophic* (thinned skin) and *hypertrophic* (thick skin) scarring. Scars can be counted and even precisely quantified with special cameras and measuring devices. But what about acne's negative emotional effects and potential damage to the psyche? Active acne in the here and now, pigmentation problems from where acne was, and the emotional effects from acne in the past all can take their toll.

ACNE CAN SCAR BOTH THE SKIN AND THE PSYCHE

Acne can exert a very serious short- and long-term emotional toll on the person suffering with this difficult condition. Acne scars can last a lifetime and have deleterious effects in all areas of a person's life. Work, school, and social, emotional, and sexual functioning can be negatively affected by the occurrence of acne. This is not new news. In 1948, Sulzberger and Zaidens stated in a definitive textbook of dermatology that "there is no single disease which causes more psychic trauma, more maladjustment between parents and children, and more general insecurity and feelings of inferiority, and greater sums of psychic suffering than does acne vulgaris" (669). A recent study reported that as many as 40 percent of dermatology patients with acne reported associated psychological problems, including clinical depression, suicidal thoughts, and low self-esteem (Gupta and Gupta 2001b). Another study, published in the *Archives of Dermatology*, found that adult acne sufferers reported a lower quality of life due to their acne than did younger patients with acne (Lasek and Chren 1998).

It is important for you to understand that the so-called objective severity of acne does not necessarily predict the emotional impact on the affected person. Put another way, what you see is not necessarily what you get. I have seen patients with very mild acne, only a few small blackheads on the chin, who will not leave the house nor participate in social activities. In contrast, I have seen patients with very extensive acne who seem to feel little serious emotional impact. Therefore, no one but you can determine how your acne makes you feel. It is our obligation as health-care providers to look through your eyes, to appreciate and respect your emotional reactions, and to design effective interventions to improve your skin and quality of life.

EMOTIONAL HAVOC: THE CAPRICIOUS NATURE OF ACNE

One of the most troubling aspects of acne is its capricious occurrence. Simply stated, it appears to come whenever it chooses. Although some acne is predictable (premenstrual, occurring at the time of ovulation, stress-induced, and so on), most acne emerges in an unpredictable fashion. Moreover, it often occurs at the most unwelcome times.

Capricious occurrences in your life can be the source of excitement, welcome variety, and great joy or, in the case of unwanted happenings, the source of significant anguish and distress. Human beings need a sense of control and some degree of mastery over their environment. This is evident in the desire of young children to repeat the same song or activity over and over. They delight in their ability to predict and control outcomes. This need for control and predictability carries over into adulthood and throughout your life.

The unpredictable nature of acne and the seeming inability to control it leaves many people in a state of psychological disequilibrium. Many studies have documented that acne causes human suffering and misery. Anxiety, depression, anger, social withdrawal, impaired school and work performance, diminished interpersonal and intimate functioning, and impoverished self-image are all documented consequences of acne (Gupta and Gupta 1998; Jowett and Ryan 1985). Thus, a crucial goal in treating acne is to give you better control over the occurrence and severity of your outbreaks.

WHAT CAN WE DO ABOUT ACNE

The bottom line is that there are two main problems that need to be fixed. The first problem is the hair follicle lining cells that have become abnormally sticky. These cells must be made normal again so they can be released and shed from the follicle rather than forming plugs that clog the follicle. Once this is accomplished, acne lesions will disappear, and new pimples will be prevented from forming. Without clogged pores, no P. acnes is trapped, and the entire cascade leading to inflammatory acne is prevented.

The second problem is the potentially destructive inflammation that occurs at the level of the hair follicle. This inflammation is due to both local and more generalized (whole-body) immune reactions to *P. acnes* trapped in the hair follicle. For mild acne, treatments must be effective at decreasing inflammation at the level of the hair follicle. If you have more inflammatory acne (bigger or deeper red and tender bumps), treatments must be effective at decreasing the more generalized overzealous immune and inflammatory reactions. Chapter 4 will describe in detail the available and emerging treatments that can address these problems and work to "fix" the broken follicle.

■ Susan

So what happened with Susan? You may think I am about to give you a happily-ever-after ending. Well, here's the story. Susan arrived at my office with a huge shopping bag filled with over-the-counter products she had purchased from the Internet, in spas and salons, and from Home Shopping Network. She had skin cleansers, toners, astringents, spot gels, pore strips, detoxifying masks, vitamins, colon cleansers, and nutritional supplements. In total, she had spent over three thousand dollars. She was confused and overwhelmed, and she had no logical or structured skincare regimen. She often found herself randomly grabbing a bottle and applying or scrubbing in desperation. Areas of excessive oiliness seemed to overlap with areas of dryness. Irritation, flaking, and skin sensitivity plagued her daily.

Our professional relationship began with her tearful explanation of her journey to my office. I assured her that her story was a common one and that I understood how difficult and traumatic adult acne can be. Then, I briefly explained the reasons for adult acne and reassured her that her acne could be well controlled. I asked that she abandon (at least temporarily) her over-the-counter products and use only the products I recommended. I prescribed a brief course of oral antibiotics combined with topical medications. The regimen was quick and simple, and it allowed Susan to wear whatever makeup she desired. Her skin responded quickly.

Susan's anxiety and sadness were so pervasive that she felt unable to continue in her job. At my suggestion, she began biofeedback therapy and cognitive behavioral psychotherapy, and she was able to continue functioning well at work. Her acne did improve and eventually subsided. Perhaps most interestingly and importantly, Susan began to rearrange her priorities. She was extremely dedicated to and successful at her job. In fact, she was so dedicated that it left her little or no time for personal endeavors. She occasionally dated, but work deadlines and commitments always seemed to interfere with relationships. Susan had often said, "Romance is clutter that inevitably leads to unnecessary messes, so why get involved?"

Well, the humbling experience of adult acne proved to also be a liberating experience. Living with extensive acne forced Susan to challenge her rigidly held belief that hard and all-consuming work and self-discipline could keep everything in order. Cognitive behavioral therapy helped her to examine her thought patterns (including her need for perfection above all else) and reorder her priorities by examining her needs for meaningful human contact and recreation. Biofeedback training taught her specific techniques for stress reduction. Susan became more socially interconnected and began exploring hobbies and leisure interests. Work remained important, but it became one facet of her life rather than her definition of her life. She inadvertently stumbled into some "clutter" and married him. She is now pregnant with her first child and has wondered aloud whether her affliction was in fact a blessing in disguise.

TAKING A CLOSER LOOK: HOW HAS ACNE AFFECTED YOU?

It can be very helpful for you to complete a brief self-test to determine what role acne is playing in your life. Many people find this test enlightening because it can shed light on effects that usually go unnoticed. Even more intriguing is the fact that this test can pick up effects exerted by acne from the past. In other words, you need not have active acne now to be suffering from the effects of acne. The good news is that this can be a starting point to gather data that can be used to improve the quality of your life.

Make a few photocopies of this exercise so you can take the test again in the future.

EXERCISE 1.1:   THE ACNE INTRUSION SCALE

This test is a series of statements. Rate each statement by circling a number from 1 (does not describe you at all) to 7 (absolutely describes you). You cannot pass or fail this test, so simply be honest.

1. As a result of having acne or acne scarring, I am uncomfortable and anxious when socializing with my friends.

    not at all true   1   2   3   4   5   6   7   definitely true

2. As a result of having acne, I find it difficult to go to work.

    not at all true   1   2   3   4   5   6   7   definitely true

3. As a result of having acne, I feel self-conscious.

    not at all true   1   2   3   4   5   6   7   definitely true

4. As a result of having acne, I feel angry.

    not at all true   1   2   3   4   5   6   7   definitely true

5. As a result of having acne, I often feel anxious.

    not at all true   1   2   3   4   5   6   7   definitely true

6. As a result of having acne, I am often moody.

    not at all true   1   2   3   4   5   6   7   definitely true

7. As a result of having acne, I feel tired and lethargic.

    not at all true   1   2   3   4   5   6   7   definitely true

8. As a result of having acne, I feel unattractive.

    not at all true   1   2   3   4   5   6   7   definitely true

9. As a result of having acne, I find that I avoid dating situations.

   not at all true   1   2   3   4   5   6   7   definitely true

10. As a result of having acne, I am not interested in sex.

    not at all true   1   2   3   4   5   6   7   definitely true

11. As a result of having acne, I am not self-confident.

    not at all true   1   2   3   4   5   6   7   definitely true

12. As a result of having acne, I feel like I don't have control in my life.

    not at all true   1   2   3   4   5   6   7   definitely true

13. As a result of having acne, I am dissatisfied with my body.

    not at all true   1   2   3   4   5   6   7   definitely true

14. As a result of having acne, it is difficult for me to exercise.

    not at all true   1   2   3   4   5   6   7   definitely true

15. As a result of having acne, I find that I drink alcohol to excess.

    not at all true   1   2   3   4   5   6   7   definitely true

16. As a result of having acne, I feel unproductive.

    not at all true   1   2   3   4   5   6   7   definitely true

17. As a result of having acne, I feel pessimistic.

    not at all true   1   2   3   4   5   6   7   definitely true

18. Because I have acne, my significant other is not interested in me.

    not at all true   1   2   3   4   5   6   7   definitely true

19. Because I have acne, being a parent is more stressful than it would otherwise be.

    not at all true   1   2   3   4   5   6   7   definitely true

20. Because I have acne, my life is not as good as it could be.

    not at all true   1   2   3   4   5   6   7   definitely true

21.   As a result of having acne, I am not likely to try new things.

not at all true   1   2   3   4   5   6   7   definitely true

22.   As a result of having acne, I tend to over- or undereat.

not at all true   1   2   3   4   5   6   7   definitely true

23.   As a result of having acne, I am generally stressed.

not at all true   1   2   3   4   5   6   7   definitely true

24.   As a result of having acne, I don't like to be touched.

not at all true   1   2   3   4   5   6   7   definitely true

25.   As a result of having acne, I find that I often pick at my skin.

not at all true   1   2   3   4   5   6   7   definitely true

Score: _____

Now add up all the numbers you circled. If you scored 75 or more, it is very likely that acne has had some negative impact on your life. A score of 100 or more suggests that acne is substantially affecting your quality of life. A score of 125 or greater suggests that acne is taking a great toll on your quality of life and you may be suffering from clinical depression. If you scored above 125, I suggest you consider seeing a therapist and take one of the many simple screening tests for depression. Many safe and effective treatments for depression are available.

This information can be a wonderful wake-up call for you. It may well be time to further examine your thoughts and feelings about your acne and yourself. Recognizing and effectively challenging your negative thoughts can positively affect your mood and skin. Using the exercises provided in this book can be a great start at regaining happiness and feeling more in control of your acne. Later in the book, you will have the opportunity to explore more about the role that acne plays in your life. I will suggest simple, positive exercises to help you take action to improve the quality of your life.

I will ask you to refer to this test periodically as you read the book. Reviewing the questions can help you clarify how acne is affecting your life. After you have practiced some of the exercises, retake the test. I expect that you will see a reduction in the negative impact of your current or past acne. If you feel that your life is really miserable or you have any active thoughts of hurting yourself or anyone else, I urge you to contact a mental health professional or your primary care doctor immediately. These sad or miserable feelings can always be made better with appropriate intervention.

2

Basic Skin Care for Acne

Acne-prone skin is the skin of betrayal. Look at all the love, attention, and money it gets. You work so hard to take care of it and spend so much money on products for it—the least it could do is behave. This chapter is meant to be practical. I want you to spend your time and money wisely.

WHEN IT COMES TO SKIN CARE, SIMPLE IS BEST

Please recall that acne is rarely the result of poor hygiene. Because many acne sufferers feel dirty, they often find themselves engaged in extensive rituals designed to get the skin clean enough so they will no longer suffer from acne. These attempts to clean or even sterilize the skin often cause more problems than they solve. Overzealous cleansing of the skin can lead to irritation of both normal skin and acne lesions. Excessive irritation of acne lesions can potentially create such a vigorous inflammatory response that scarring can occur. Irritation of normal skin can break down the normal epidermal barrier, allowing irritants, allergens, and infectious agents (bacteria, fungi, and viruses) to enter the skin. The result is often angrier skin, more acne, and even serious infection.

So, why is there so much hype about skin cleansing regimens for people with acne? Well, it is partly based in the myth that acne is a disorder of inadequate hygiene. The other factors sustaining the belief in elaborate skincare regimens may be related to the profit motives of manufacturers.

The Basics: General Skin Care

The best skin care need not be costly nor enormously time consuming. Your skin needs only gentle cleansing in order to remove dirt and skin debris, unless your occupation or hobby coats the skin with grease, oil, paint, or other difficult-to-remove substances. While you may prefer the feeling, your skin need not sting nor feel tight in order to be very clean. In fact, if your face doesn't feel very dry after you wash it, the product you used is probably a good one for your skin.

OILY SKIN

If your skin is oily, gentle use of a toner, astringent, or clarifier should be more than sufficient to cleanse the skin. These products are designed to remove skin oil and soap film and can be applied with the fingertips, cotton balls, or soft, nonabrasive pads. I recommend choosing a toner, astringent, or clarifier that is alcohol free.

Although it's not strictly necessary, you may choose to use a cleanser also. If you do, select one that is gentle and noncomedogenic, such as Neutrogena Oil-Free Acne Wash. Cleansers are best applied to a wet face with warm water, using the fingertips to gently massage the skin.

Some dermatologists recommend products with herbal ingredients based on the belief that they are gentler. I am not convinced that they are necessarily gentler, and allergic reactions to herbal products are often seen in our practice.

DRY SKIN

If your skin is dry or very sensitive, you should avoid toners and astringents as well as drying or heavily scented soaps. Use of a nonsoap, low-alkaline replenishing cleanser such as Neutrogena, Cetaphil, Oil of Olay, or Aquanil can be helpful. Cleansers with glycerin are good for people with normal and dry skin, since they don't remove the invisible lipid layer that is the face's natural protective film.

COMBINATION SKIN

Most of my patients tend to have combination skin. They are oily on the nose, the area adjacent to the nose, and the forehead (the T-zone), while they are typically drier on the cheeks. I recommend slightly more vigorous cleansing or use of toners and astringents in the oily areas, with more gentle care for the drier areas. Gentle cleansers such as Cetaphil, Neutrogena, and Oil of Olay products for sensitive skin can be excellent choices.

Using Acne-Fighting Products

While I do stand by my statement that in general, elaborate skincare routines are unnecessary for good hygiene and healthy skin, combinations of acne-fighting products are often needed to control acne. If you are using over-the-counter skincare products, they probably contain ingredients such as benzoyl peroxide, salicylic acid, and glycolic acid. Prescription products also often contain these ingredients, used in combination with topical antibiotics and topical retinoids (I'll discuss these in more detail in chapter 4). These preparations can potentially be both drying and irritating to the skin. Therefore, you should take care to avoid using overly drying cleansers at the same time, since they can increase your likelihood of experiencing skin irritation. Using nonsoap cleansers and cleansers with glycerin can be a better choice if you are using other acne-fighting products that contain benzoyl peroxide, salicylic acid, or glycolic acid. Dermatologists commonly assess your skin type to ascertain your degree of oil production and the sensitivity of your skin. This type of skin evaluation allows for an appropriately chosen blend of products that will be maximally effective with minimal irritation.

The Myth of the Moisturizer

I am sure that you have been told that moisturizers clog your pores and cause acne. Well, just when you were getting over your disappointment that there is no such thing as the tooth fairy, here comes another hard-to-swallow fact: Moisturizing the skin does not cause acne. As long as the skin is gently cleansed, applying moisturizing products will not make your acne worse. This is a terrific thing, since many acne products are drying, and you often need the balancing effects of a moisturizer to avoid excessive dryness, flaking, and irritation.

ACNE AND SUNSCREENS

Acne sufferers frequently experience more breakouts during the warmer months, when sunscreen is more liberally used. Therefore, sunscreens are often vilified as acne-causing agents. In reality, the ingredients in sunscreens are probably not very *comedogenic* (acne causing).

There are two general classes of sunscreens: those that contain chemical agents that bind to molecules inside the skin to provide sun protection and those that contain physical agents that remain on top of the skin, forming a barrier that prevents penetration of the sun's rays.

Chemical sunscreens typically contain some combination of avobenzone (Parsol 1789), oxybenzone, methoxycinnamate, octocrylene, octisalate, homosalate, or octyl salicylate. The *physical sunscreens* usually contain either zinc oxide or titanium dioxide in a micronized form. In other words, they are pulverized to such tiny particles that they are almost invisible to the naked eye. The chemical agents can be more irritating and are more likely to cause allergic reactions of the skin. The physical agents are less irritating, and allergic skin reactions are more rare. However, physical sunscreens may prompt more sweating beneath them, and thus they can potentially promote more acne, *folliculitis* (irritation of the hair follicle), and *miliaria* (prickly heat). Many newer sunscreens combine both chemical and physical blocks, allowing for greater protection. Therefore, the possibility of irritation, allergy, and *occlusion* (covering or blocking) is real for most available sunscreens.

So, do sunscreens cause or at least contribute to acne? Maybe, but their antiaging and anticancer benefits clearly outweigh any acne-forming effects. Their potential to cause acne can usually be minimized by good product selection and good skin care. Gels are generally better choices for acne-prone skin, since they are more drying and less occlusive. Gentle cleansing of the skin before initial application and reapplication can be helpful. I must stress that the products available for daily use, such as moisturizers with sunscreen, have minimal potential for occlusion and irritation. The issues discussed above are largely applicable to the dedicated sunscreen for use at the park, pool, or shore. I urge you not to abandon your use of sunscreen in the pursuit of clear skin. Skin cancer, deep wrinkles, dark brown spots, rough texture, and sagging skin can produce even worse scars than acne.

CONTACT IRRITATION

Clothing, sweatbands, athletic equipment, or other skin adornments that occlude or rub the skin can cause and aggravate acne. Under occlusion, perspiration is trapped along with bacteria. Both can irritate and gain entry into the hair follicle. Pretreating the skin with an antiacne product and gently washing as soon as possible after significant perspiration can be helpful. Wearing loose-fitting, absorbent clothing can also be helpful.

ACNE AND THE SEASON

If you live in an area where winters are significantly drier than summers, I am sure that you have noticed that your skin's needs change with the season. Skin tends to be drier in the winter and more oily in the summer, and the humidity in the air seems to intensify the oiliness. Skincare products that are more drying and potentially more irritating—such as toners, astringents, clarifiers, alpha and beta hydroxy acids, and benzoyl peroxide preparations—are better tolerated and even welcome in the summer. In contrast, the low ambient humidity of the winter months often leaves the skin thirsty for moisture, making less drying and better moisturizing acne care products more desirable.

PREVENTING AND CARING FOR ACNE ON THE CHEST, BACK, AND BUTTOCKS

Acne in places other than the face generally occurs for the same reasons as acne on the face. However, as you already intuitively know, the opportunities for occlusion and irritation are greater in these locations due to clothing, friction, and perspiration. Treatment regimens are essentially the same as for facial acne, with a few caveats. Washes are often easier, since the involved body surface area is usually greater. Backs and buttocks can usually withstand higher-concentration and more drying antiacne products without irritation. In contrast, the chest is often more sensitive and can therefore become irritated and develop rashes more easily. The possibility of occlusion as a cause or worsening factor should always be considered. Loose-fitting cotton garments can be helpful, and pretreating acne-prone areas before dressing and before exercise is recommended.

Using medications in these covered areas can be problematic, frustrating, and expensive. For example, benzoyl peroxide preparations can bleach and discolor clothing. Some of my patients have had favorite shirts ruined in this manner. Other topical products can rub off and also discolor clothing. Therefore, using leave-on products on the chest, back, and buttocks may be best done at night, recognizing that sheets and pillowcases can suffer similar discoloration. Morning treatments of these areas are best limited to shower washes, thin nonstaining lotions, or no treatments at all.

Sometimes, the face and the body respond differently to treatment. You may find that the chest and back are the last areas to respond, or you may find just the opposite. Moreover, some treatments that clear the face will be ineffective for the back, and vice versa.

Keep in mind that in the realm of skin care, simpler is almost always better. I'll discuss treatment of acne in detail beginning in chapter 4, but for now, you know the basic principles of good skin care.

3

Targeting Your
Acne Triggers

One of the most distressing aspects of acne is its apparently arbitrary nature. Breakouts simply seem to happen whenever they feel like it, without any rhyme, reason, or predictability. While there is some truth to this, it's also true that you can learn to identify what triggers some of your acne and modify those triggers to help prevent breakouts. The exercises in this chapter will guide you in beginning the process of gaining control of your acne—and your life.

IDENTIFYING YOUR ACNE TRIGGERS

With the help of some good sound detective work, triggers for some of your breakouts can be identified. Moreover, monthly and seasonal patterns can sometimes be identified. Understanding these patterns and triggers can have two benefits. The first is that you may avoid or modify the acne triggers, and this may result in fewer and less severe breakouts. The second benefit is that of knowledge and predictability. When you know why your breakout has occurred, how severe it is likely to be, and roughly how long it will last, you will feel more in control and better able to make treatment and lifestyle choices. This will reduce some of the seemingly constant uncertainty you live with as an acne sufferer. For example, if you reliably break out more during the middle of your menstrual cycle or during the week before your period, increasing your use of topical and oral acne treatments before these breakouts occur may significantly reduce the extent of the breakout. If stress and anger seem to be triggers, practicing a stress reduction exercise or positive self-talk exercise (these are included later in the book) may prove helpful in both reducing acne and improving the quality of your life.

I want to reiterate that despite the claims made by acne know-it-alls, "one size fits all" generalizations regarding what caused your acne and how to fix it are invariably wrong. The factors that altered your hormones or your follicular response to your hormones are unique and specific to you. The list of possibilities and "maybes" can be overwhelming. Absolutes offered by friends and relatives (such as *Change your diet, Sleep more, Change your cosmetics,* or *Drink more water*) may not have any relevance to you. Even more confusing is the fact that what caused yesterday's breakout may be different from what caused your breakout last week.

I would like you to begin this important task of better understanding your acne by completing the Acne Trigger Identifier exercise. This initial assessment is intended to help you recognize general patterns and triggers for your breakouts. An acne trigger is anything that appears to cause you to have more pimples, to develop angrier pimples, or to pick or otherwise manipulate your pimples. Taking notice of these triggers can enable you to make specific changes that may well improve your acne.

I encourage you to occasionally refer back to this Acne Trigger Identifier exercise. You may find that your perceptions regarding each of the potential triggers change as time goes by. Scientifically, we know that multiple sampling almost always gives more accurate information. Thus, each time you take this assessment, you will gather more meaningful information about your acne. You'll generate acne management information that is specific to you and your physiology. Overall, you can come to a better understanding of what contributes to your breakouts, and you will feel better knowing that you have more control over how your skin behaves.

EXERCISE 3.1: ACNE TRIGGER IDENTIFIER

Complete this simple exercise by checking yes or no in pencil.

I seem to break out more the week before my menstrual period.	☐ Yes	☐ No
I seem to break out more at or soon after the onset of my period.	☐ Yes	☐ No
I seem to break out more when I am feeling stressed.	☐ Yes	☐ No
I seem to break out more midcycle (around the time of ovulation).	☐ Yes	☐ No
I seem to break out more when I wash my face less often.	☐ Yes	☐ No
I seem to break out more when I use styling gel in my hair.	☐ Yes	☐ No
I seem to break out more when I wear more makeup.	☐ Yes	☐ No
I seem to break out more when I am feeling angry.	☐ Yes	☐ No
I seem to break out more when I am eating more milk products.	☐ Yes	☐ No
I seem to break out more when I am eating more carbohydrates.	☐ Yes	☐ No
I seem to break out more when I am sleep deprived.	☐ Yes	☐ No
I seem to break out more when I am not exercising regularly.	☐ Yes	☐ No
I seem to break out more when I am exercising more.	☐ Yes	☐ No
I seem to break out more when I pick at my face.	☐ Yes	☐ No
I seem to break out more when I have a cold or flu.	☐ Yes	☐ No

In the space provided below, list the factors you have identified that appear to elicit or worsen your acne or cause you to pick at or otherwise manipulate your acne.

Factors that appear to worsen my acne:

_____

_____

_____

_____

_____

By reviewing and analyzing your answers to the questions in this exercise, you have probably discovered some very useful information about your skin and what makes it more reactive. Based upon this information, I strongly encourage you to examine aspects of your life and lifestyle that seem to be related to your acne and begin to consider some changes that could be helpful for you and your skin.

Remember, your goal is to generate useful data that is as precise and specific to your individual body chemistry as possible. In the pursuit of this goal, let's get even more personal and specific. I would like you to fill out a daily record of your breakouts to refine the data that you have already generated. Make enough copies of the Daily Acne Log (exercise 3.2) to last for three to four weeks. At the end of each day, check the word that best describes your acne for that day: mild, moderate, or severe.

Observe your diet. Is it high carbohydrate or low, high or low in fat, high or low in partially hydrogenated oils? Record all medications, vitamins, and herbal medicines and the amount of water intake. Also record the types and amount of cosmetics used. Rate your level of stress, anger, fatigue, and happiness as low, medium, or high. Exercise issues include the frequency and regularity of workouts and time until showering. Also make a note of the clothing worn (tight-fitting spandex, headbands, and so on). Illnesses such as colds, flu, or infection should be noted. Women can chart the time of month either as day one (signifying the first day of your period) through day twenty-eight (the last day before your next period) or simply as after period, midcycle, or premenstrual. Please record anything else that seems even remotely relevant in the "Other" space. Sometimes, events that seem far removed from the skin can affect your acne.

The Daily Acne Log can be an invaluable tool, allowing you to specifically identify and track the factors in your life that aggravate your acne. I strongly encourage you to carefully and thoughtfully use this daily log; the benefits may exceed your expectations.

EXERCISE 3.2: DAILY ACNE LOG

Date: _____

Today, my acne was   □ mild   □ moderate   □ severe

Diet: _____

Medications: _____

Vitamins/herbal medicines: _____

Water intake: _____

Cosmetic use: _____

Stress level: □ low   □ medium   □ high

Anger level: □ low   □ medium   □ high

Level of fatigue: □ low   □ medium   □ high

Overall feelings of happiness: □ low   □ medium   □ high

Exercise: _____

Clothing: _____

Illness: _____

Time of month: _____

Other: _____

I hope that the Daily Acne Log has helped you identify even more specific information about what appears to aggravate your skin and trigger your acne. Don't be discouraged if the patterns you have identified are inconsistent. I am absolutely convinced that there are times when acne simply happens for no apparent reason. However, discovering and modifying your triggers can make a very large difference in the frequency and severity of your outbreaks. Allow me to tell you about Frank, one of my tough customers.

■ Frank

Frank came to see me with a four-year history of very stubborn acne that had been treated with numerous topical preparations and oral therapies, including isotretinoin. He was able to clear about 80 percent of his acne lesions, but only while taking high doses of oral antibiotics and using very irritating topical medications. I suggested to him that perhaps stress and other lifestyle issues might be contributing to the stubbornness of his acne and his need for ongoing oral antibiotics. His eye roll and obvious annoyance at my suggestion made his position clear. Frank believed that anything other than pills and creams was bogus. Rather than argue with him, I simply told him that the choice was his: continue on his present regimen of antibiotics, with no end in sight, or try something new. My nurse handed Frank copies of the Acne Trigger Identifier and Daily Acne Log. Frank promptly stuffed them into his pocket.

I suppose you think that I am going to tell you that as soon as Frank began using these assessment tools, he had an immediate and spectacularly positive response. Nope. What happened was a much more gradual change. Frank did identify several important triggers for his acne. He found that sleeping less than seven hours, eating numerous very high carbohydrate meals, and high stress made him break out more. Not only did stress worsen his acne, it also increased his tendency to pick at his skin. Finally, Frank—like many people—noted that he reliably broke out more when under significant stress at work.

So, the bottom line was that the Acne Trigger Identifier and Daily Acne Log did prove helpful for Frank. Let's look specifically at how he used the information to change his lifestyle.

First, Frank made a concerted effort to more regularly get seven hours of sleep. Movies and books were the biggest culprits, so he promised himself he would try to shut off the movie or close the book at a reasonable hour. When seven hours of sleep was not possible, Frank made a conscious effort to control other triggers such as diet and stress. He was careful not to become overly concerned if a party, a worry, or the needs of his wife or kids kept him from getting the coveted seven hours of sleep. The important goal was a more global one of better managing the collection of lifestyle factors, not controlling every one, every day.

Second, Frank looked for a reasonable balance in his diet. If he had a meal loaded with carbohydrates, he would look to balance that meal with good protein sources and healthy fats at other times during the day. He realized that his previous diet had placed his body on a bungee cord, yanking him forcefully to extremes. He had noticed that his excessive intake of carbs was always followed by severe, punitive, self-imposed sugar restrictions. His physiology and emotions often were similarly affected, with highs and lows throughout the day. Now, he felt more even-keeled and generally happier. It was all about avoiding extremes. He felt less stressed as he envisioned his body and skin receiving a steadier and more healthful supply of essential nutrients.

Third, Frank learned stress management techniques. He set a goal to listen to a guided imagery relaxation tape for ten minutes at bedtime. He also made a conscious effort to better control the intensity of his stress responses during the day. Rather than pick at his skin when feeling stressed, he would use controlled rhythmic breathing and refocus his attention elsewhere. He found that he felt less stressed overall and definitely manipulated his skin less.

Sometimes, despite his best efforts and intent, he would still pick his skin during very stressful periods. Frank realized how important it was that he avoid falling into the trap of the lost cause. Alcoholics Anonymous teaches its members about this trap. It goes like this: A person has been sober for three months. In a moment of weakness, he has a drink. This is the turning point. He can say to himself, "You see, I am an incorrigible and hopeless drunk, and a total failure. All is hopeless. I might as well finish the whole bottle in front of me." A much healthier alternative is to say, "I am sorry that I had this lapse in control, but look how well I have been doing. I will not let this small stumble jeopardize all the hard work and meaningful progress I have made thus far."

And so it is for managing stress and avoiding manipulation of the skin. Episodic picking of the skin need not lead to feelings of futility and a return to extensive skin picking. It is the sum of your responses to stress that determines how you do, not any given isolated response. The only exception to this rule is behaviors that could permanently harm yourself or others. These behaviors cannot be part of your repertoire of options in response to stress or anger.

Frank's realization that most of his inflammatory breakouts occurred during times of increased stress allowed for a change in his antibiotic regimen. Frank and I agreed that he should take his oral antibiotic only during periods of increased stress, when he felt his skin was more prone to breakouts.

These lifestyle changes had a very substantial and positive effect on Frank's life. Over a three-month period, his acne improved to the point that only a topical retinoid cream and alpha hydroxy acid lotion were necessary to maintain good skin. He would still get occasional cystic outbreaks, but they responded quickly to oral antibiotics, usually within two to three days. Moreover, Frank felt much happier and less stressed in his life.

Good for Frank, but more importantly, what about you? Let's take a look at how you can use the information you've gathered to make changes that will improve your complexion.

MODIFYING YOUR ACNE TRIGGERS

I encourage you to review your Acne Trigger Identifier and Daily Acne Log. Based on this information, make a short list of goals consisting of lifestyle factors you wish to modify. These goals should be very specific. Vague statements of desired changes (such as I *should exercise more, eat better, be less stressed*) inevitably fail because they provide no measurable markers of progress and success. Spell out your desired changes in concrete terms. For example:

- I will get seven hours of sleep five nights a week.

- I will exercise three times a week for twenty minutes.

- I will practice my stress reduction exercises ten minutes per day.

- I will not leave my makeup on overnight.

- I will reduce my intake of carbohydrates and refined sugars to a certain number of grams per day. (Current recommendations suggest that carbohydrates should make up approximately 50 to 60 percent of your total dietary intake. They should be complex carbohydrates with a low glycemic index—those that don't produce rapid and extreme rises in blood sugar; for example, vegetables, whole-grain breads, and brown rice.)

You may choose to work on reducing your inner tension and stress by meditating once or twice daily or using the other stress reduction techniques discussed in chapter 8. If you are a picker, you should plan alternative behaviors that you can do when you have the urge to pick. You can carry worry beads or a stress ball, do finger stretch exercises, make tea, or chew gum. Basically, engage in any alternative activity that will focus your attention away from your skin and break the repetitive cycle of skin picking.

Make several copies of the Acne Trigger Modifier Plan (exercise 3.3). In all likelihood, you will modify this plan several times in the future. Again, be specific regarding your goals for any of the areas you choose. Start a new Acne Trigger Modifier Plan each week.

EXERCISE 3.3: ACNE TRIGGER MODIFIER PLAN

Date:

Diet:

Exercise:

Stress management:

Cosmetic use:

Medication use:

Skin manipulation:

Other:

KNOWLEDGE IS POWER: UNEXPECTED HEALING BENEFITS

Many people find a substantial number of unexpected benefits after using the program for several weeks. The benefits are best described as both skin and life enhancing. Previously unrecognized patterns of behavior become obvious. They are literally "in your face" as you look at your Acne Trigger Identifier and Daily Acne Log. Acne-aggravating and otherwise unhealthful behaviors are difficult to ignore with your heightened awareness. I often hear from my patients that they find themselves seeking out and engaging in healthier activities as a result of what they've learned. Knowledge is power. Even better, knowledge with specific tools and techniques for change has the power to enhance and heal.

Healing is a main thrust of this book. Healing acne lesions and healing the physical and emotional scars left by acne is your goal. Healing is possible for everyone, but it is often a slow process. Don't become discouraged if you do not see immediate and dramatic improvements in your skin and your overall sense of well-being. Often, very meaningful changes are happening that are beneath the skin and away from your awareness, creating better health for your body and skin.

Most likely, you will find that the techniques offered in this book will enable you to effectively modify your acne triggers, behaviors, and stress reactions. It is possible, though, that you may become aware that anxiety, stress, inner tension, or compulsive behaviors are usurping more of your emotional and physical energy than you wish. If the self-help techniques you learn in this book do not bring the level of improvement you need, then professional counseling—alone or together with antidepressant or antianxiety medications—is often very helpful.

4

Skin Treatments for Acne and Acne Scarring

You are now quite knowledgeable about the true origins of acne. You realize that due to a collection of genetic, hormonal, and environmental factors, pimples develop because of abnormalities of the pore lining cells that result in clogging of the pores. Unfortunately, these clogged pores provide a dark, oil-rich environment that allows *P. acnes,* the bacteria that causes acne, to flourish. In addition, inflammation caused by substances released by this trapped bacteria—and the body's immune response to the bacteria-laden pore—leads to red, inflamed acne. Unchecked, this process can lead to scarring. In this chapter, I'll discuss common acne treatments, including treatments for existing pimples and for scars from acne.

Before getting started with the specifics of treatment, I would like you to consider this introductory caveat: If it sounds too good to be true, it is probably too good to be true. I urge you to beware of quick-fix guaranteed success and 100 percent satisfaction guarantees. As you learned in the last chapter, the available over-the-counter formulations are ineffective for many acne sufferers. The false claims about these products pave a path of broken promises. These broken promises and less-than-optimal results understandably lead people to become frustrated and skeptical. They therefore abandon treatment and fail to seek out legitimate medical therapies.

Remember that acne is not a simple disease. There is a complex series of events that leads to the formation of acne lesions, and that process cannot be reversed overnight. Simple, miraculous "cures" are impossible. Each person's skin and acne is different. The exact causes of your acne may be very different from the causes of the acne your friend has, even thought hers looks just like yours. Therefore, the treatment that works marvelously for her may be a disaster for you. Adult acne, by definition, lives on skin that has had more years of sun exposure and wear and tear than teenage skin. Your more mature skin may be less tolerant of some of the very drying and irritating products commonly used for teenage skin. Home remedies, over-the-counter products, stress management techniques, and herbal therapies work very well for some but poorly for others. Prescription medications and treatments tend to work better and faster and are often used together with the nonprescription remedies. Over-the-counter and natural therapies are not necessarily safer for the skin or your body. These treatments often undergo no Food and Drug Administration testing for safety, purity, and lack of allergic reactions.

The good news is that almost everyone's acne can be well controlled with the proper therapies. Thus, take heart that if one treatment does not work well for you, another surely will. There is virtually no one whose acne cannot be brought under good control by modern medical and complementary therapies.

COMMON ACNE TREATMENTS

Trying to sort through the acne products on the drugstore shelves alone can be confusing. Then, adding to these products the blur of remedies offered in magazines, on television, and on the Internet, the choices become overwhelming. Near total chaos can occur when prescription products are added to the mix.

You are on the road to becoming an educated and empowered consumer. Understanding how each product works and why you are using it will make you much more successful in improving and managing your acne. In this section, I'll provide a straightforward and useful road map of acne treatments that separates treatments into general categories based upon how the products work. The categories are as follows:

- treatments that normalize pore lining cells

- treatments that kill bacteria

- treatments that decrease inflammation

- treatments that *exfoliate* (remove) dead skin cells, helping to unclog pores

- treatments that decrease oil gland production

- treatments that alter hormones or hormone effects

- lasers, ultraviolet, and intense light therapies

- herbal and vitamin therapies

I will briefly discuss each of these treatments and provide you with some common names of the products that are included in each category. Rarely is a single agent effective for adult acne. Combination treatments are much more effective and are usually necessary to achieve substantial improvement.

Acne products are often available in washes, solutions, gels, lotions, creams, and ointment formulations. Washes are quick and often used at the sink or in the shower. They can be mildly drying but rarely cause significant irritation. Gels and solutions tend to be more drying and less greasy; thus they are best for oily skin. Lotions are in between, while creams and ointments are more moisturizing and therefore best for dry, sensitive skin. Ointments can be fairly greasy, limiting their desirability in the morning and under makeup. If you have very dry skin, an ointment formulation applied at night followed by a lotion, cream, or solution in the morning may work best.

Treatments That Normalize Pore Lining Cells

This important category mainly involves *retinoids,* which are vitamin A–based medications that work to improve acne by normalizing follicular lining cells (preventing the clogging of pores) and decreasing inflammation. The American Academy of Dermatology has recently stated that retinoids are considered an essential component of the treatment regimen for all acne types: blackheads, whiteheads, and inflammatory acne (Gollnick et al. 2003). Topical retinoids are prescription products and include tretinoin (Retin-A, Renova, Avita), adapalene (Differin), and tazarotene (Tazorac). Retinoids keep the pores open, so pimples do not form and *P. acnes* does not flourish. They are used to both treat and prevent acne. The newest topical retinoid product, Velac, is unique because it is a combination product containing tretinoin (the active ingredient in Retin-A) and clindamycin (a commonly prescribed antibiotic). (At press time, Velac was awaiting FDA approval.)

A tantalizing additional benefit of retinoids is their antiaging properties. They have been proven to have stimulatory and normalizing effects on the skin. *Collagen* is a protein in the middle layer of the skin that is responsible for the resiliency of the skin. Collagen, which normally decreases and fragments with sun exposure and age, is actually increased in quantity and normalized by topical retinoids. The melanocytes, which are the pigment-producing cells in the skin, often over-produce melanin as we age, leading to brown spots. These are also normalized by retinoids. Clinical benefits include reduction in fine wrinkles, improved skin texture, and lightening of brown spots. Another benefit of topical retinoids is that the skin often feels smoother and looks more vibrant, and people report that makeup applies more evenly and easily.

The problem with retinoids is that they can be drying and irritating. People vary in their skin response to retinoids. Some are able to use retinoids twice daily, while others can use them only twice weekly. Most people find that with regular use of retinoid products, these nuisance side effects occur less often. I specifically refer to them as "nuisance" side effects because many people mistakenly interpret any irritation or redness as a sign of allergy or other adverse reaction. This can result in discontinuation of the medication, an unfortunate choice since retinoids are so important for both acne management and rejuvenation of the skin.

Contrary to popular misconceptions, retinoids do not thin the skin. The top layer of the skin, which is composed of dead skin cells waiting to slough off, is smoothed and slightly thinned by retinoids. All living layers of the skin, which thin with age, are actually restored to normal thickness. The modest sun sensitizing effects of retinoids are due largely to the thinning of the top dead skin layer.

The retinol in over-the-counter products differs from that in prescription retinoids in that it is not yet actually an active medication. In order to become effective as an antiacne or antiaging product, retinol must first be converted to its active acid, retinoic acid, by enzymes in the skin. There are only a limited number of these enzymes in the skin. Therefore, only the higher concentrations of retinol, such as 0.3 and 0.5 percent, are considered to have substantial effectiveness. The reason is that the higher the concentration of retinol in the product, the more available and active the retinoic acid that is formed.

In contrast, Retin-A, Renova, and Avita are already retinoic acids that require no additional conversion to be effective. More retinoic acid is available to normalize the follicular lining cells and promote healing of the skin. Thus, in general, these prescription products are more effective in treating acne than are most over-the-counter retinol products.

ISOTRETINOIN

The queen of all normalizers is *isotretinoin*. This oral retinoid is without a doubt the most effective acne treatment available today. It normalizes follicular lining cells, decreases inflammation, and decreases oil production. For most people, it essentially "fixes" acne, at least for a while. It reverses the skin abnormalities that cause acne, leading to acne-free skin in the vast majority of people treated. So what is the catch? If it is so effective, why isn't everyone simply treated with isotretinoin?

First and foremost, oral vitamin A preparations such as isotretinoin can cause birth defects if taken during the first trimester of pregnancy. This effect occurs only if you are taking the medicine while pregnant. Oral retinoids have no effect on resting eggs, ability to become pregnant, ability to carry to full term, nor your ability to have a fully normal child after discontinuing isotretinoin. Since isotretinoin has been available for more than twenty years and more than 20 million people have taken the medicine, its safety with regard to childbearing—provided it is not taken *during* pregnancy—has been proven in two generations of use.

The second issue centers on a question about a possible link to depression and suicide. Over the years, there have been occasional reports of depression and even attempted and actual suicides in isotretinoin users. This must be balanced by the recognition that acne itself is an independent risk factor for depression and suicide. Further, these reports often were based on adolescents, who by definition have a high incidence of depression (at least 10 percent). In the United States, 3,500 to 4,000 young people commit suicide each year (Sadock and Sadock 2001).

At the time of this writing, numerous studies have addressed this issue. In summary, the link appears weak at best. The occurrence of depression and suicide in people taking isotretinoin does not exceed that seen in an age- and sex-matched group in the general population (Jick, Kremers, and Vasilakis-Scaramozza 2000). Further, two studies have shown that isotretinoin can actually make depression better (Rubinow 1987). This is not surprising, since living with acne can literally be depressing. As acne disappears, so can the related depression.

The common side effects of isotretinoin are dose related and usually very mild. Since vitamin A dries the skin and mucous membranes, dry skin and dry lips are the most common complaint. These effects are usually easily managed with moisturizers, lubricants, lip gloss, and lip balms. Other side effects—including fatigue, joint pain, decreased night vision, hair shedding, and elevation of cholesterol and triglycerides in the blood—are less common and usually seen with higher dosages. If you are on isotretinoin, take care to use good sun protection and avoid waxing of the skin for hair removal. The medication can make you more sensitive to the sun, and the skin can be more fragile during treatment. Aggressive laser procedures should also be avoided while you are taking isotretinoin.

Treatments That Kill Bacteria

Numerous topical products are effective at decreasing the amount of bacteria on the skin and in the follicle.

BENZOYL PEROXIDE

Benzoyl peroxide is an excellent *antimicrobial* (bacteria-killing) agent and is the active ingredient in many over-the-counter products, including Oxy, Persagel, Panoxyl, and many generic drugstore brands. The level of benzoyl peroxide usually ranges from 2.5 to 10 percent. The higher concentrations are sometimes more effective but can be drying and irritating. Despite the fact that benzoyl peroxide products can be irritating to the skin, they actually have some anti-inflammatory effects as well. Therefore, they can be helpful in reducing the inflammation surrounding the hair follicle. If your skin is oily, you probably will tolerate higher concentrations and appreciate the drying effects. If you have drier, more sensitive skin, lower concentrations and preparations mixed with moisturizing agents will be required.

Different formulations of benzoyl peroxide are available, including washes, gels, pads, and creams. The washes are commonly used at the sink or in the shower, while the creams, pads, and gels are used at night or in the morning before application of moisturizer, sunscreen, or makeup. Brevoxyl, Triaz, and Zoderm are excellent prescription benzoyl peroxide preparations available in a variety of strengths and formulations. Over-the-counter benzoyl peroxide products (Oxy, Persagel) are often recommended for prevention and treatment of mild to moderate acne. They are often used alone but sometimes are formulated together with salicylic acid or glycolic acid. Prescription products often combine benzoyl peroxide with clindamycin (BenzaClin or Duac) or erythromycin (Benzamycin) in order to increase effectiveness and reduce the development of resistant bacteria.

SALICYLIC ACID

Salicylic acid is another common ingredient in over-the-counter formulations that has reasonably good antibacterial and anti-inflammatory activity. Similar to benzoyl peroxide formulations, salicylic acid products are available in washes, gels, and creams. Clearasil, SalAc, Clean & Clear, and Salex are common examples.

TOPICAL ANTIBIOTICS

Topically applied antibiotic preparations are effective in killing *P. acnes*. Common examples include erythromycin (Aknemycin, T-Stat pads), clindamycin (Clindagel, Clindamax, Cleocin T), and sodium sulfacetamide with and without sulfur (Klaron, Rosac, Rosanil, Ovace, Rosula). These products should be used in combination with other topical antiacne products to minimize the development of resistant strains of bacteria. Velac, a topical combination product containing a retinoid (tretinoin) and an antibiotic (clindamycin) was awaiting FDA approval at press time. The tretinoin will help to keep the follicle open and less likely to trap *P. acnes*. Dapsone, an antibiotic previously available only in oral form, is presently being developed for topical application. Topical dapsone (Aczone) may prove helpful in treating acne due to its antibiotic and anti-inflammatory properties.

Topical products are always preferable when possible, since any oral medication can be associated with allergic or other adverse reaction. An advantage of using topical antibiotic preparations is their negligible absorption into the blood. Therefore, there is no alteration in the normal balance of bacteria and fungi in the body.

ORAL ANTIBIOTICS

Sometimes, topical preparations are not sufficient to control acne despite regular use and good skin care. Oral antibiotics such as doxycycline (Adoxa, Doryx, Vibramycin), minocycline (Dynacin, Minocin, Vectrin, Myrac), and erythromycin (E.E.S., Eryc, Ery-Tab) are more effective in killing bacteria and also have anti-inflammatory properties. Oral antibiotics, while certainly more effective than topical therapies, can have a variety of side effects, including sun sensitivity, gastrointestinal upset, and vaginal yeast infections if you are predisposed. As with any oral agent, a host of nuisance and serious side effects can occur.

The growing problem of antibiotic-resistant bacteria is a serious one. The liberal and widespread use of powerful, *broad-spectrum* antibiotics (those capable of killing most bacteria in our environment) is fostering the development of new strains of bacteria. MRSA (methicillin resistant staph aureus) is being increasingly seen in communities throughout the US. This infection was previously confined to hospitals. If the rate at which these resistant bacteria develop outpaces the ability of the pharmaceutical industry to develop new antibiotics capable of killing them, we are all in big trouble.

The antibiotics used by dermatologists to treat acne are usually narrow-spectrum, weaker agents that are effective at killing *P. acnes* and also effective at decreasing inflammation in the skin. They should always be used together with topical agents to minimize the development of resistant strains of *P. acnes*.

Despite the fact that there is data to support the safety of these antibiotics for the long-term management of acne, I believe that you should always be looking for an exit strategy. If you are on one of these oral antibiotics, regular attempts to reduce your dosage or discontinue the medication should be made. You should also review with your physician the other existing and new treatments that are available.

SUBANTIMICROBIAL-DOSE DOXYCYCLINE

A new approach that is effective for many acne and rosacea sufferers is Periostat, a very low-dose oral doxycycline preparation. Periostat is considered a *subantimicrobial* product because it does not kill bacteria; rather, its mechanism of action is based on its powerful anti-inflammatory effects. Since it does not kill bacteria, the natural balance of bacteria and fungi remain unaltered in the body, and theoretically, it cannot foster the development of resistant bacteria. Extensive microbiology testing has been performed to ensure that Periostat has no antibiotic properties. Periostat benefits the acne and rosacea patient by inhibiting the inflammatory cascade of effects of *P. acnes*. Periostat may also benefit people with *comedonal* (whitehead/blackhead) acne. In view of the real and growing issue of bacterial resistance, this treatment regimen is an exciting addition to our existing acne and rosacea treatments. Periostat can also be useful as a maintenance medication for people who have previously relied on antibiotics for long-term acne control.

Treatments That Decrease Inflammation

Inflammation is responsible for red bumps and red, tender pimples, and it also can lead to scarring. Therefore, controlling inflammation is a crucial part of acne treatment. As you learned earlier this chapter, topical agents such as retinoids, benzoyl peroxide preparations, and salicylic acid products all demonstrate some anti-inflammatory properties. Oral antibiotics (including doxycycline, minocycline, and erythromycin) are even better anti-inflammatory agents in addition to having antimicrobial effects. Several newer agents directly address the inflammation associated with acne and may prove useful as complementary or add-on agents for controlling acne. One promising new development involves the use of topical immune modulators, either alone or in combination with retinoids and antibiotics.

NICOMIDE

Nicomide (nicotinamide or niacinamide) is a recently introduced product with some data to support anti-inflammatory and antiacne activity. Nicotinamide is an antioxidant and a free radical scavenger, meaning that it functions to neutralize damaging by-products of both normal and abnormal cellular reactions. Nicotinamide also appears to inhibit the release and activity of other potentially damaging chemicals. Nicotinamide is one of the two principal forms of the B-complex vitamin niacin (the other is nicotinic acid).

Nicomide is available as a gel and as pills. The pills also contain zinc oxide, cupric oxide, and folic acid, which may enhance the effectiveness of nicotinamide as an anti-inflammatory. Side effects of topical nicotinamide can include irritation and occasional stinging.

ELIDEL

Elidel (pimecrolimus) is a nonsteroidal anti-inflammatory cream approved for the treatment of *eczema,* an inflammatory condition of the skin. Elidel is not currently approved for the treatment of acne. However, since Elidel is steroid free, it can be used topically as an anti-inflammatory without fear of damaging and thinning the skin. Elidel works by inhibiting the activation of certain immune cells in the skin and may have some benefit for controlling inflammatory acne characterized by small red bumps. Elidel may be of some benefit by itself, but it is probably most useful when mixed with potentially irritating medications such as topical retinoids and benzoyl peroxide. Combining Elidel with these products may decrease or eliminate skin irritation. Elidel appears to have few side effects other than occasional stinging on application. Elidel is a topical immune suppressing cream, and therefore there is a theoretical possibility of increased skin infection or malignancy. Neither of these adverse effects have been seen in clinical use.

DIETARY CONSIDERATIONS

The role of diet in acne is controversial. Most well-controlled scientific studies do not support a connection between what you eat and the presence or absence of acne. There are some diet advocates who believe that consumption of processed sugars, saturated fats, and hydrogenated oils contribute to acne. A 2005 study in the *Journal of the American Academy of Dermatology* (Adebamowo et al.) found a link between teenage acne and dairy intake. The authors speculate that the observed association is due to the presence of hormones and other biological substances in milk. Rather than avoiding milk (an excellent source of protein and calcium), a more prudent approach may be drinking organic milk from cows free of hormone-supplemented feed.

Essential fatty acids receive a great deal of attention from nutritionists and herbalists and are often recommended to help acne. These fatty acids are called "essential" because they must be obtained through diet; the body can't make them. The body converts some essential fatty acids into the hormonelike substance *prostaglandin*, which reportedly has anti-inflammatory effects on the skin. Herbalists believe some people with acne lack enough essential fatty acids in their diet. Gamma-linolenic acid (GLA) is an effective anti-inflammatory that is limited in human diets. It is alleged to help keep hair, skin, and nails healthy. GLA is available in certain dietary supplements. Borage oil is the richest source of GLA. Black currant seed oil and evening primrose oil are also good sources of GLA. Omega-3 fatty acids appear to be beneficial in decreasing systemic inflammation and may possibly have some complementary effect when combined with standard medical therapies for people with inflammatory acne (Logan 2003). These fatty acids are found in salmon, mackerel, fish oil capsules, flaxseed, and flaxseed oil.

A few studies have found deficiency in linoleic acid in the skin of acne patients. However, they were not found to be otherwise deficient in this essential fatty acid. Oral supplementation was not substantially beneficial. Boone and Pierard (1998) found that topical application of linoleic acid resulted in a 25 percent reduction in *microcomedones* (the earliest acne lesion). The role of linoleic acid in treating acne remains controversial.

Treatments That Exfoliate and Unclog Pores

Since clogged pores are a key factor in the development of acne lesions, removing dead skin cells and unclogging the pores is an important approach to treatment. This can be achieved using alpha hydroxy acids, beta hydroxy acids, or microdermabrasion.

ALPHA HYDROXY ACIDS

Alpha hydroxy acids (AHAs) are naturally occurring organic acids such as glycolic acid (a natural constituent of sugarcane juice) and lactic acid (found in sour milk and tomato juice). They are topically applied agents that increase the rate of cell turnover, decrease the stickiness of cells, and exfoliate the skin. As a result, the compacted layer of dead skin cells is made thinner and smoother, and the opening of the pore is less likely to be clogged. These actions can be beneficial in treating and preventing some types of acne (blackhead, whitehead, and mildly inflammatory acne). Dermatologists offer in-office AHA peels in concentrations ranging from 20 to 70 percent. Glycolic acid is the most common type of peel. Home peeling products have recently become available from major cosmetic companies. Their efficacy for treating acne has not yet been established.

BETA HYDROXY ACIDS

Beta hydroxy acids (BHAs) such as salicylic acid can produce similar benefits. AHAs and BHAs also have been shown to have rejuvenating effects on the skin. They stimulate production of collagen, improve the texture of the skin, reduce fine wrinkles, and lighten areas of increased pigmentation. These treatments can be done at home with washes, lotions, and creams or more intensively with peels performed in a medical or salon setting. The "beta lift" is a common salicylic acid peel performed in a medical office.

The main difference between alpha hydroxy acids and beta hydroxy acids is their ability to dissolve in oil. Alpha hydroxy acids dissolve in water only, while beta hydroxy acids can dissolve in oil or water. This difference suggests that theoretically, beta hydroxy acids are better able to penetrate the oil-rich hair follicle to promote exfoliation. Despite this theoretical advantage, AHAs and BHAs are probably equally beneficial for acne.

Both AHA and BHA peels can be helpful for blackhead/whitehead acne and small red bump acne. The peels are useful to treat the acne lesions themselves and can also hasten the resolution of postacne pigmentary problems. Peels performed in physicians' offices are usually much stronger and more effective than those performed in nonmedical settings. The cost can range from $75 to $250 per peel. In order to achieve significant results, the peel regimen typically consists of a minimum of four to six peels, spaced at two- to four-week intervals. Side effects are generally mild, and immediate return to work is usually possible. This is why these treatments are sometimes called the "lunchtime peel." Modest redness lasting for the duration of the day of the peel is expected. Mild superficial skin peeling lasting several days is commonly seen with BHA peels. Occasionally, intense redness and blistering can occur. Scarring from these peels is exceedingly rare if they are performed properly. At-home use of topically applied creams, lotions, and washes can also be of some benefit, but the results are slower and more modest.

MICRODERMABRASION

Similar acne and antiaging benefits can be achieved from microdermabrasion (Dermagenesis, Dermapeel, Power Peel). *Microdermabrasion* is a procedure during which a suction tip gently lifts the skin while fine sterile particles are used to polish and exfoliate the superficial layers of the skin. The combination of suction and gentle exfoliation easily removes dead skin and debris. Blackheads often disappear as they are removed from the impacted follicle. Benefits include acne improvement, improvement in acne scars, smoother skin texture, improvement in fine wrinkles, and the reduction of unwanted hyperpigmentation. Microscopic studies have documented improvements in the skin, including increased collagen production, which is considered concrete proof of rejuvenation. There is mild stinging during the procedure, similar to the sensation you would experience walking into the wind on a very windy day at the beach. Side effects are usually very mild and include redness and mild skin irritation typically lasting for only one day. Occasionally, a raw patch or even a scab occurs.

Similar to alpha hydroxy acid peels, microdermabrasion yields much more impressive results when performed with a medical-grade system under medical supervision, rather than with a less powerful salon-grade system. Four to eight sessions are usually necessary to achieve reasonable benefit.

Microdermabrasion is a very different procedure than traditional dermabrasion. Traditional dermabrasion is a very aggressive process that abrades off the top layer of the skin and a portion of the middle layer of the skin. There is very substantial downtime and significant discomfort. Dermabrasion is not used for the treatment of active acne but can be useful for treating acne scars.

Treatments That Decrease Oil Production

Unfortunately, there are really no topical agents that dramatically decrease oil production. However, long-term use of topical retinoids may slightly decrease oil production. Microscopic studies of the skin have shown some decrease in the size and oil production of the sebaceous gland as a result of topical retinoid use. Oral isotretinoin is effective in decreasing oil production but carries risks that frequently outweigh the benefits. Other approaches are available that decrease the amount of oil on the skin. These include astringents, toners, oil control gels, and blotting papers.

ORAL ISOTRETINOIN

Oral isotretinoin dramatically decreases oil production by the sebaceous gland, creating a less favorable environment for *P. acnes*. Due to the other issues surrounding isotretinoin (birth defects if used during pregnancy, rare effects on blood lipids, and occasional reports of depression and suicide), it is not FDA approved for the decrease of oil production.

Low-dose isotretinoin regimens are enticing because both oil production and acne occurrence can be decreased. When isotretinoin is used in low doses, the severely dry skin, muscle aches and pains, and even hair loss that can occur with higher dosing regimens are rarely seen. However, there are potential problems with low-dose regimens of isotretinoin. To begin with, while longer-term use at low doses is probably safe, there are not well-controlled clinical studies looking at this treatment regimen in the general population of acne sufferers. Further, if pregnancy is even a remote possibility, the longer you are on the medication, the greater the chance of an unintended pregnancy. Then there is the question of duration. How long do you stay on the medication? Will prolonged treatment with low-dose isotretinoin give lasting freedom from acne and decreased oil production once the medication is stopped? Since the answers to these questions are unknown, it is probably unwise to use isotretinoin solely for the purpose of oil control.

ASTRINGENTS AND TONERS

Astringents and toners remove excess skin oil and dry the skin. They have no effect on oil production. Therefore, by drying the skin at the beginning of the day with an astringent or toner, it will take longer for the oil being produced to accumulate on the skin and become evident.

OIL CONTROL GELS

Oil control gels (Clinac OC) contain microscopic sponges that soak up skin oil and invisibly flake off when the skin is washed. Like toners and astringents, oil control gels don't have any effect on the rate or amount of oil produced by the skin. These gels can allow you to get through the day without skin oil seeping out through your makeup.

OIL BLOTTING PAPERS

Oil blotting papers absorb oil and remove it from the skin. These can be helpful since you can use them without removing your makeup first. They are pressed or blotted on the skin, and oil is absorbed without significant effect on the makeup.

Treatments That Alter Hormones or Hormone Effects

Geneticists, anthropologists, and psychiatrists are sometimes quoted as saying that biology is destiny. Well, the truth with regard to acne is that if you inherit acne-prone skin as part of your biology, then we can say testosterone is destiny. Once adult hormone production begins at puberty, it is largely testosterone that is responsible for initiating the process of acne formation in predisposed people. Therefore, effective hormonal treatments either decrease testosterone production, dilute or decrease its concentration in the blood, or block the testosterone receptor so that it cannot stimulate the pore.

THE ORAL CONTRACEPTIVE PILL

The *oral contraceptive pill* (OCP) is frequently touted as a great treatment for acne. In reality, it can be helpful for some but not all acne sufferers. Certainly, the OCP is not an option for men. The OCP is usually an estrogen-based product such as ethinyl estradiol combined with a progesterone product such as norgestimate (Ortho Tri-Cyclen) or drospirenone (Yasmin). These products dilute testosterone by adding estrogen to the blood, and they also increase a protein (sex hormone binding globulin) that binds testosterone, making it unavailable to stimulate the hair follicle to cause acne. The OCP is usually fairly well tolerated, but common side effects can include bloating, nausea, breakthrough bleeding, weight gain, and mood changes. Often, switching to a different OCP will eliminate or minimize these effects. Anyone with a personal history of breast cancer, blood clots, or migraine headaches is not a candidate for the OCP. The overall safety of the OCP has been a subject of debate in recent years, and decisions regarding its use should be made carefully after discussion with your health-care provider. The most recent studies on the risks and benefits of the OCP suggest that there may be a very slight increase in the relative risk of breast cancer, while the risk of ovarian and endometrial cancer is decreased by 50 percent (Taylor 2005).

SPIRONOLACTONE

Spironolactone (Aldactone) is a medication that works very differently than the OCP. Essentially, it blocks the ability of testosterone to stimulate the abnormal cell changes in the hair follicle that lead to acne. Spironolactone is mainly used as a *diuretic* (water pill) for a variety of medical conditions where the body retains too much water. It can be helpful for acne because it binds to the testosterone receptor on the hair follicle but does not activate it. Therefore, testosterone is unable to bind to the follicle because the "parking spot" is already occupied.

Much like the OCP, spironolactone is not effective for everyone. It often is used together with the OCP. This combination therapy tends to work better, and side effects such as midcycle breakthrough bleeding and breast tenderness that are seen with spironolactone alone are less common. Spironolactone rarely causes elevation of blood potassium, but blood levels of potassium must be periodically checked. Abnormalities are extremely rare if your kidney function is normal. While spironolactone is believed to be safe in humans, very high doses in animals can be associated with breast tumors.

I would like to share with you a final cautionary point. I tell each and every one of my patients that any time a medication, vitamin, herbal preparation, or food passes your lips, an *idiosyncratic reaction* (individual hypersensitivity) is possible. This means that while a given reaction may be very rare, anything is possible: rashes, nausea, vomiting, diarrhea, liver or kidney effects, blood count effects, and psychiatric effects. Put another way, you must consider whether the pain of the problem is greater than the pain—or the potential pain—of the solution.

Laser Treatments for Acne

Borrowing from a religious reference, show me the light and I will show you the way. Lasers are often portrayed as the miracle light that will erase skin imperfections and fix the damage of the "sun sins" of the past. Initially, studies were conducted using a visible light source (blue light) with the hope of inactivating *P. acnes*. The results were hopeful but not overly impressive. As is true for many medical discoveries, the discovery that lasers could be effective for treating acne was largely serendipitous. A 1,450-nanometer laser called the Smoothbeam was being used to treat wrinkles and acne scars without any thought or intent that it might be effective in treating or preventing acne. To their pleasant surprise, both physicians and a good percentage of patients who were being treated with this laser noticed a substantial improvement in the patients' active acne. These unexpected effects were reported in the dermatology literature, and a tidal wave of interest and enthusiasm ensued.

Clinical and microscopic studies have shown that the Smoothbeam laser inactivates bacteria and changes the sebaceous gland in a favorable way, leading to decreased acne. Studies are now under way using other laser wavelengths and intense light sources, some in combination with new topical medications, to inactivate *P. acnes* and improve acne. Needless to say, just about every company that manufactures a laser, intense pulse light, or other medical light source is now investigating the effectiveness of their product for the treatment of acne. Stay tuned, since this laser miniseries is far from over. While these therapies are believed to be safe, the short- and long-term risks and benefits remain to be seen.

Photodynamic therapy is a variation of light and laser therapy. This treatment, which is not yet FDA approved for the treatment of acne, uses a topically applied medication called ALA (aminolevulinic acid; brand name Levulan Kerastick). A short time after application of the medication to the skin, a laser or other light device is used to activate the medication. The laser- or light-activated medication generates *free radicals*, metabolic chemicals that are toxic to *P. acnes* and reduce the activity of the sebaceous gland. Preliminary studies have shown improvements in acne (Gold 2005).

Complementary Therapies

Practitioners of complementary and alternative medicine often recommend herbal and vitamin therapies to treat acne. These practitioners do not necessarily reject traditional medical treatments but rather augment them with herbs, supplements, and other therapies. Americans spend large sums of money on complementary and alternative medicine, with annual estimates approaching $29 billion (Trattner 2002).

Evaluating the effectiveness of herbal therapies is extremely difficult. Topical products such as tea tree oil, aloe vera, green tea extracts, alpha lipoic acid, zinc, selenium, and vitamins A, B, C, and E are often sold with claims of spectacular all-natural therapeutic effectiveness. The problem is that unlike in some European countries, where herbal therapies are more widely accepted by the government and practitioners, herbal and other natural therapies in the United States are often not held to any legal standards to ensure safety and effectiveness. Controlled clinical studies comparing these products to those with no active ingredient are also typically not done. In short, there is very little current data showing that these therapies are as effective as—or any safer than—the traditional over-the-counter or prescription products.

Despite this, cosmetic companies such as Neutrogena, Estée Lauder, and Procter & Gamble have actively embraced the societal enthusiasm for herbal products, adding ingredients such as soy, allantoin, chamomile, DMAE, tyrosine, alpha lipoic acid, green tea extract, glutathione, cucumber extract, l-ascorbic acid, cimicifuga racemosa extract, and hyaluronic acid to some of their products.

I am not at all opposed to herbal and vitamin therapies if you have found them helpful, either as your only skin therapy or as additions to traditional acne therapy. In fact, I frequently recommend products containing green tea extracts and vitamins A, B, C, and E for their anti-inflammatory and antioxidant actions. A few prominent dermatologists will recommend oral supplementation with vitamin A (8,000 IU daily) and zinc (80 mg daily).

THE RATIONALE BEHIND COMPLEMENTARY THERAPIES

In theory, products that possess anti-inflammatory and antioxidant properties should decrease inflammation in the skin. Further, products that may decrease *sebum* (skin oil) production and favorably alter the hair follicle response to testosterone should have some antiacne benefits. There is convincing data that green tea polyphenols and vitamin C act as anti-inflammatory agents and free radical scavengers (Draelos 2005). Microscopic and biochemical studies have proven this to be true. More importantly, clinical benefits in real life have been observed in the skin. Topically applied vitamin C has been shown to decrease the redness of the skin in people who suffer from rosacea, and there have been case reports of effectiveness in improving acne. Vitamin E is essential for vitamin A (which maintains healthy skin and hair follicle cellular activity) to function normally.

VITAMIN-BASED TREATMENTS

Niacinamide, the active form of vitamin B_3 (niacin), is receiving a good deal of attention. It has anti-inflammatory, antipigmentation, and antiacne effects. Both topical and oral preparations are now available. It appears helpful for treating problems with pigmentation, since it suppresses the transfer of *melanin* (pigment) to the skin surface.

Vitamin B_5 (pantothenic acid) is involved in human fat metabolism and may have some effect on sebum production in the skin. A Chinese study (Leung 1995) utilizing both oral and topically applied pantothenic acid found decreased sebum production and fewer inflammatory acne lesions. Proponents of pantothenic acid as a treatment for acne recommend 100 mg orally daily.

Vitamin B_6 (pyridoxine) is involved in the metabolism of steroid hormones. Deficiency of pyridoxine in animal studies led to increased sensitivity of the sebaceous glands to testosterone (Snider and Dieteman 1974). Since testosterone is one of the "evil" hormones implicated in acne, increased sensitivity to testosterone is certainly something to avoid. Some practitioners have recommended vitamin B_6 supplementation at 100 mg per day orally.

MINERAL-BASED TREATMENTS

Zinc is considered an essential mineral for protein and collagen synthesis. It also functions as an anti-inflammatory and has regulatory effects on testosterone and vitamin A function. Interestingly, zinc may inhibit 5-alpha reductase, the enzyme that converts testosterone to DHT, a potent androgen that causes male pattern baldness and increases sebum production. While controlled studies of efficacy are lacking, some practitioners recommend 25 to 100 mg of zinc orally daily to acne sufferers. Topical application of zinc may increase the effectiveness of benzoyl peroxide and erythromycin preparations, but efficacy studies are contradictory.

Selenium is a trace mineral that has anti-inflammatory properties and aids the body in utilizing vitamin E. Selenium deficiency has been occasionally noted in female acne sufferers, thus complementary medicine practitioners will sometimes recommend 100 to 200 μg daily, to be obtained from foods and supplements. Caution must be exercised, since long-term intake of too much selenium (more than 400 μg daily) can produce unwanted side effects such as brittle nails and hair loss. Food sources of selenium include tuna, Brazil nuts, whole wheat, garlic, broccoli, and brown rice.

HERBAL TREATMENTS

Herbs such as chamomile can be soothing to the skin, but care should be taken, since some people experience irritation or allergic reactions to both natural and synthetically derived skin care products. Chamomile contains alpha bisabolol, which has been demonstrated to have healing and anti-inflammatory properties.

Topical application of tea tree oil has been shown to have some anti-inflammatory, antioxidant, and antimicrobial effects and in theory could be helpful for acne. A small study (Bassett, Pannowitz, and Barnetson 1990) demonstrated effectiveness similar to benzoyl peroxide, with less irritation.

Green tea polyphenols enjoy the reputation of being powerful antiaging and protective agents. Topical application to the skin has shown anti-inflammatory and antioxidant effects and provides some protection against ultraviolet damage. They may have an inhibitory effect on 5-alpha reductase, thereby potentially decreasing sebum production. Syed and Zulfiqar (2001) compared 2 percent green tea extract cream to a placebo cream. The active cream group had a 75 percent reduction in acne lesions, while the placebo group achieved only a 7 percent reduction.

Soy phytoestrogens are a group of plant compounds that have estrogenlike effects. There is some evidence that they increase skin thickness, inhibit skin pigmentation, and may have some blocking effects on androgens (Baumann 2001). A small study (Liu et al. 2001) demonstrated some effectiveness of soy-containing skincare products against acne.

ISOLUTROL

Isolutrol is found in the liver and gallbladder of sharks and may inhibit oil production in the skin. Dunlop and Barnetson (1995) compared the effectiveness of isolutrol to 5 percent benzoyl peroxide. Both treatments were found effective against inflammatory lesions, but isolutrol lacked efficacy in decreasing blackheads and whiteheads. However, isolutrol did cause less irritation and dryness than benzoyl peroxide.

I have several reservations about recommending isolutrol. Widespread use of shark organ products could further jeopardize species of sharks that are endangered. Moreover, the data is insufficient to suggest that isolutrol is more effective or safer than currently available treatments.

TREATING EXISTING PIMPLES

Simply sitting back and helplessly watching a new pimple grow on your face is a miserable feeling. As I have stated elsewhere in the book, you need to feel a sense of control over your life and your acne. Thus, a question I frequently hear from my acne patients is, "What can I do when I feel a new pimple coming?" The answer depends on how aggressive you wish to be.

Physical Treatments

Physical treatments of pimples generally consist of application of cold or hot compresses, squeezing, extraction, pore strips, and injection.

COLD AND HEAT

Several acne experts believe that application of cold, such as rubbing an ice cube on the spot for a few minutes several times a day, reduces swelling and redness. Some also believe that the hydrating effects of water on the skin as the ice melts may increase the penetration of previously applied topical medications. Warm compresses do little to reduce inflammation but may decrease the force necessary to evacuate the follicle when squeezing or performing extraction on pimples.

SQUEEZING

Squeezing pimples is something that many if not most acne sufferers have done. Most dermatologists recommend against any manipulation of all acne lesions, including blackheads, whiteheads, papules, pustules, cysts, and nodules. The rationale against manipulating pimples is that scarring and worsening of the acne lesion is always a possibility. Dermatology textbooks provide graphic and troubling photographs of massive inflammation, swelling, damage to blood vessels, and scar tissue from squeezing pimples. These potential consequences must be balanced against the short-term distress of leaving the house with a pointed pus bump on the face.

If you must squeeze a pimple, I suggest that you gently cleanse the area with alcohol and use a washcloth to apply moist heat with gentle pressure for several minutes. Then, using a gauze pad or facial tissue, gently apply pressure on either side of the lesion with your index fingers. Once the pus or blackhead has been expressed, immediately stop squeezing. Additional manipulation only leads to more inflammation and possible extrusion of bacteria into the skin, both of which increase the likelihood of scarring.

EXTRACTION

Comedone or *comedo extractors* are specially designed metal instruments that allow for application of focused and symmetrical pressure to the follicle. These are the instruments used by dermatologists and aestheticians for extraction. There is some controversy within the field as to whether this type of acne surgery is in the patient's best interest. There is no doubt that sustained use of a topical retinoid preparation is a gentler and ultimately more effective treatment, since it will prevent formation of new lesions. However, retinoids take several weeks to exert their positive effects on the skin. Additionally, there are some lesions that do not respond to topical retinoid therapy and therefore must be manually removed. While the general public can obtain comedone extractors, they should be used cautiously, since overzealous use can scar the skin.

PORE STRIPS

Pore strips are cloth strips impregnated with a glue-type substance that theoretically will adhere to and pull out blackheads as the strips are pulled off the skin. They can be of some benefit, but caution must be exercised, since they can be irritating to the skin. The nose tends to be more tolerant of this method of blackhead removal, while the cheeks, chin, and forehead are sometimes more sensitive. If you are using topical retinoid preparations, you should be especially careful, since retinoids can increase skin sensitivity.

INJECTIONS

Injection of a dilute corticosteroid solution directly into an inflamed acne lesion can have a dramatically positive effect, with rapid decrease in size, redness, and tenderness. Actors and actresses and others who are frequently in the public eye will often avail themselves of this treatment. While it is dramatically effective, there are potential pitfalls, including loss of pigmentation and development of a sunken area at the site of injection. Injection of acne lesions should only be performed by dermatologists or other appropriately trained professionals.

Topical Treatments

Spot gels containing salicylic acid, benzoyl peroxide, sulfur, and sulfur-resorcinol blends can speed the resolution of pimples. There are literally hundreds of these products available. Examples include Neutrogena Advanced Solutions Acne Treatment, Neutrogena Rapid Clear Acne Eliminating Gel, Oxy 10 Emergency Spot Treatment, Johnson & Johnson Persagel, Bioré Blemish Double Agent, and

Clinique Acne Solutions Emergency Gel. Summers Laboratories makes several agents that contain some camouflage makeup, such as Rezamid, Loroxide, and Liquimat. These treatments are certainly not as dramatic as an injection but can shorten the duration of an outbreak by several days.

Application of prescription acne products such as Differin, Retin-A, and Tazorac in addition to spot gels can be of some benefit. A few experts will occasionally recommend topical corticosteroid preparations. Only high-potency prescription formulations are helpful, though, and drawbacks include the possibility of skin thinning, loss of pigment, and excess blood vessel formation. Occasionally, oral ibuprofen at 1,200 mg per day has been recommended, but its effectiveness has not been demonstrated other than in one small study (Wong, Kang, and Heezen 1984).

TREATMENT OF ACNE SCARS

While one of the main goals of effective acne treatment is to avoid scarring of the skin, sometimes treatment is begun too late or simply fails to prevent scars from forming. If you have scars on your face from acne, please take heart, because there is much that can be done.

■ Rebecca

Rebecca, a patient new to my practice, sobbed quietly with tears of joy when I told her that her scars could be improved without intrusive or life-threatening interventions. At the age of forty-two, she had spent the last twenty years free of active acne but burdened by the innumerable small indentations on her cheeks. She last saw a dermatologist fifteen years before, at which time she was told that full-face dermabrasion under general anesthesia was her only option. She was told that the procedure was painful and invasive, with significant potential for additional scarring and infection. Needless to say, that sounded like an unappealing prospect.

Treatment of Rebecca's scars with the Smoothbeam laser, combined with microdermabrasion, gave her about a

60 percent improvement with essentially no downtime. Rebecca was very pleased. She felt her complexion was smoother overall and the scars generally less obvious. This was enough improvement for her, and she found a greater sense of freedom with her newfound attractiveness.

I cannot emphasize strongly enough that evaluation and treatment of acne scars is a bit of a tricky business. Acne lesions leave scars of many types, each requiring a different treatment approach for improvement. Therefore, treatment of acne scars requires evaluation by a skin specialist with extensive experience in this area. While there is some disagreement regarding the ideal treatment for each type of acne scar, experts generally agree that

- different types of acne scars require different treatments in order to achieve good results,

- deeper scars usually require more aggressive treatments for substantial improvement,

- the degree of improvement that can be achieved with a less aggressive scar remediation treatment varies considerably and cannot be precisely predicted for a given person, and

- complete elimination of acne scars with no telltale signs is usually not possible.

In general, the depth of the scar, the type of indentation, and the amount of obvious tissue damage overlying the scar are important factors determining the type of treatment necessary and the degree of improvement possible. I will briefly review for you the available approaches and the types of scars for which they are generally used.

Excision and Subcision

Surgical removal is often necessary for deep, ice pick acne scarring or other larger scars that are substantially bound down. *Ice pick scars* are those that appear as if the skin has been pushed deep down by an ice pick. Scars that are bound down are those that cannot be elevated, even when the skin on either side of the indentation is stretched. In both of these cases, the skin has been damaged and pulled down by extensive scar tissue formation.

Surgical *excision* of ice pick acne scars is usually done with small surgical punches exactly matched to the size of the ice pick indentation. Surgical punches are instruments that look like tiny cookie cutters or apple corers. They allow for precise removal of tissue, leaving behind a circular defect. Scars can be removed in their entirety by "punching out" and removing the entire scar.

Variations on this technique include punch elevation and punch grafting. With *punch elevation,* the skin freed by insertion of the surgical punch is not removed completely but rather elevated and sutured in place level with the surrounding skin. *Punch grafting* involves removal of the skin released by the surgical punch and subsequent replacement with skin obtained from other anatomic areas (usually behind the ear). The skin is harvested using an identical surgical punch or sometimes a slightly smaller one. Larger scars are removed by surgical scalpel. The opening or defect in the skin is then closed with fine surgical sutures. Approximately six weeks later, the surgical site may be treated with dermabrasion, microdermabrasion, or laser to minimize the surgical scar. The result is usually quite good, with a more even contour and texture of the skin.

Another possible option for some sunken scars is *subcision.* This procedure involves inserting a sterile needle into the base of a scar and attempting to manually cut the fibrous strands of scar tissue. The degree of improvement tends to be unpredictable. Substantial bruising and skin discoloration can persist for many months.

Dermabrasion

Dermabrasion is a fairly aggressive technique in which the physician uses a motorized tool with a rapidly spinning metal head or spinning fine wire brush to abrade off the top layer of the skin (the epidermis) and the upper part of the middle layer of the skin (the *papillary dermis*). The tissue damage produced by dermabrasion initiates *remodeling,* a healing process whereby new collagen is formed and thickened. The remodeled collagen can plump up sunken areas of scarring. After several weeks, the regenerated epidermis is often smoother and more normal in appearance. Needless to say, this is a procedure that requires several weeks of postoperative skin care and some downtime due to the crusty and scabby appearance of the skin.

The procedure requires a steady hand, and the depth of abrasion must be precise, or additional scarring can occur. Producing damage too deep in the *dermis* (the middle layer of the skin) can destroy the hair follicle and the sebaceous oil gland. Once these structures are destroyed, permanent scarring and loss of pigmentation can result.

Even when dermabrasion is performed properly, problems with pigmentation may result, with either over- or underproduction of pigment leading to formation of dark or light spots. Skin is sometimes treated before and after surgery with hydroquinone-based products to avoid hyperpigmentation. Rigid use of sunscreen after dermabrasion is important to avoid hyperpigmentation from the sun. Pigmentary loss is more difficult to manage. If it does occur, use of topical tacrolimus (Protopic) may help the *melanocytes* (the cells that produce pigment in the skin) to resume their pigment production. Despite these caveats, the improvement following dermabrasion can be dramatic and can parallel some of the more modern and "glitzy" procedures.

Chemical Peels

Chemical peeling of the skin is a procedure that involves precise and controlled application of an acid. Chemical peels exert their effects on the skin by destruction of the skin and by stimulating the skin. Agents such as glycolic and salicylic acid and trichloroacetic acid (TCA) are commonly used for superficial peels. These peels do minimal damage to the skin, often removing little more than the dead skin cell layer. Their modest beneficial effects on scarring appear to be based on their ability to stimulate collagen production and to increase the production of specialized proteins called *glycosaminoglycans*. In order to obtain any observable results, four to eight peels spaced from two to six weeks apart are usually necessary. The skin is likely to be pink for the remainder of the day after the peel, and small blisters may form. There is usually little or no downtime.

Deeper chemical peels can achieve greater scar improvement but require substantially greater tissue damage. These peels usually remove part or all of the epidermis. The damage and inflammation can result in collagen remodeling and regeneration of the epidermis.

The most commonly employed agent for deeper peels is trichloroacetic acid (TCA). TCA is applied to the skin in concentrations ranging from 20 to 70 percent. A common regimen is the Jessner's-TCA peel. Jessner's solution is used to cleanse the skin prior to application of the TCA, removing oil and debris and leaving the skin more permeable to the TCA. The TCA is applied and left on the skin until a whitish frost forms. The acid is then neutralized and a thick moisturizer such as Aquaphor applied. Complete skin healing takes one to three weeks. Problems with pigmentation (too much or too little) are sometimes encountered. Therefore, pretreatment and posttreatment with a retinoid and hydroquinone are common.

Phenol is sometimes used when a very deep peel is needed. While phenol peels can result in dramatic improvement, they are extremely deep peels and require substantial medical monitoring. Patients must be monitored for rare cardiac side effects. Therefore, these peels are usually performed in offices or surgery centers where an anesthesiologist is present as part of the team. In addition to the rare complications that can occur during the procedure, permanent problems with skin texture and pigmentation are possible.

An additional benefit of peels is their antiaging effects. Fine lines, rough texture, age spots, unsightly skin growths, and even precancerous growths can be eliminated.

Laser Treatments

Lasers are commonly divided into the ablative and nonablative types. To ablate means to destroy. *Ablative* lasers are those that destroy tissue, while the *nonablative* lasers theoretically are attracted only to a specific target and are not destructive to tissue.

LASER ABLATION

Carbon dioxide lasers and erbium lasers are the two ablative lasers most commonly used for skin resurfacing and scar improvement. The carbon dioxide laser burns off skin layers in a controlled fashion similar to dermabrasion but by laser energy rather than mechanical abrasion. As with dermabrasion, skin is usually removed to the level of the papillary dermis. Laser ablation has several advantages over mechanical ablation. The degree of destruction can be more precise, and there is little bleeding. The mechanism of scar improvement may be somewhat different. Laser ablation generates a great deal of heat. It is believed that heating of the collagen results in both stimulation of the collagen and scar formation in and around the collagen. These events lead to tightening of the collagen and increased collagen production. All this, together with regeneration of the epidermis, which is destroyed during laser ablation, results in scar improvement and improvement in the appearance of the skin.

Postlaser pigmentary change is a potential complication. Many people have increased pigmentation soon after the procedure, while approximately 5 percent of patients experience pigment loss nine to twelve months after treatment.

NONABLATIVE LASER TREATMENTS

Nonablative laser treatments are certainly more appealing from the patient's perspective, since there is little or no tissue destruction and virtually no downtime. The nonablative lasers most effective for acne scarring appear to be those in the 1,064–1,450-nanometer range. Usually, treatments are performed at four- to six-week intervals, with maximal benefit being seen after four to eight treatments. The degree of improvement is variable and virtually always substantially less than with the more invasive procedures. A reasonable estimate would be a 20 to 50 percent improvement at best. It is more difficult to give patients an accurate percentage of improvement that can be expected, since each person responds very differently. Similar to chemical peels, laser treatments also offer rejuvenation benefits.

Skin Fillers

Another widely used approach to the correction of acne scars is the use of skin fillers. Skin fillers can be used alone or in combination with other scar correction techniques. Fillers can plump up or elevate areas where the skin is sunken. It is important to remember that not all acne scars are amenable to this type of treatment. In contrast to the sunken scar that is bound down by extensive scar tissue, sunken scars that elevate when the adjacent skin is stretched often correct nicely with injection of skin fillers.

Ideally, skin fillers would be composed of natural, nonallergenic, affordable substances that would lead to permanent correction of the skin. Unfortunately, while filler substances continue to improve, we have not yet found the perfect filler. Fillers are divided into two broad categories: biodegradable and permanent.

BIODEGRADABLE FILLERS

Biodegradable fillers are derived from human and animal tissues. Eventually, the body metabolizes these substances and most if not all of the skin correction is lost. The rate at which the substances are metabolized depends on both the substance and the unique metabolic characteristics of the individual person.

Collagen remained the filler agent of choice up until the past few years. Collagen formulations were initially obtained from cows. Bovine collagen preparations are available in different thicknesses (Zyderm, Zyplast), each chosen according to the characteristics of the scar or wrinkle to be treated. Problems with bovine collagen include the possibility of allergic reactions, the limited duration of the benefit (three to six months), and the remote possibility of the transmission of mad cow disease.

Newer recombinant technologies have allowed for the development of human collagen preparations (CosmoDerm, CosmoPlast, Autologen). CosmoDerm and CosmoPlast are bioengineered collagen derived from human *fibroblast* cells (the cells in the skin that produce collagen). They are much less likely to cause skin reactions and theoretically can carry no risk of infectious disease. Autologen is a bioengineered collagen that is actually derived from your own tissue. It is much more expensive and requires harvesting tissue (sometimes obtained from other cosmetic procedures you may have had, including facelifts or liposuction). Artefill is a combination product designed to be a more permanent filler. It is composed of bioengineered collagen mixed with Plexiglas microbeads. While the benefits appear to be longer lasting than collagen alone, there are concerns regarding skin reactions to the Plexiglas microbeads. All collagen fillers can give good correction for certain types of acne scars. The rare allergic reactions and the short duration of the benefit are their main shortcomings.

Hyaluronic fillers have been available for several years in Europe and are the most recent addition to the filler choices. *Hyaluronic acid,* a protein, is a natural constituent of the dermis. Hyaluronic acid fills the skin by the viscosity of its own gel formulation. It also functions as a "protein sponge," attracting water and generating a matrix that further plumps the skin. Restylane, Perlane, and Hyalaform gel are currently available preparations. Hyaluronic acid appears to last longer than collagen, and skin reactions are less common. Duration of benefit is usually six to nine months but can sometimes be longer. Radiesse is a newer filler composed of calcium hydroxyapatite. Not yet approved for acne scars and skin rejuvenation, it appear longer lasting and may be beneficial. Sculptra, a newly approved filler composed of poly-L-lactic acid, is purported to last considerably longer. Used in Europe for several years, this agent appears safe except for reports of deep skin lumps. The possibility of skin reactions is being evaluated in the reformulated material available in the United States.

PERMANENT FILLERS

Permanent fillers cannot be metabolized by the body and thus should stay in place more or less permanently. The problem with permanent fillers is that they may be more likely to cause allergic reactions and rare foreign body reactions. These reactions can lead to red bumps, hard bumps, or even ulceration of the skin. As a rule, it is the older fillers and the ones promising the longest duration that are more likely to cause these reactions.

Silicone was one of the original skin fillers used for acne scars as well as other cosmetic treatments. There has been a great deal of controversy over the years regarding alleged associations between silicone and autoimmune diseases. Well-controlled studies have not supported this proposed link, but there certainly have been local skin reactions that can make silicone problematic.

Implants

A final option for the correction of acne scars is implants. These are the least commonly used techniques, but they are sometimes necessary in areas of deeply sunken skin or bound-down skin. Human tissue in the form of autologous dermal grafts or even tissue grafts obtained from cadavers can be used.

Autologous dermal grafts utilize skin harvested from a donor location on the patient's own body, usually a place where a scar will not be noticed, such as behind the ear. The dermatologist removes a piece of skin from the donor site and sutures the donor site closed. The epidermis (top layer of the skin) is removed from the dermis of the donor skin. The remaining dermis, with or without the fat below the skin, is implanted into the dermis beneath the acne scar. Permanent correction, although usually imperfect, can be achieved.

Tissues obtained from cadavers are used in a similar manner. Cadaverous sources of skin raise potential concerns about transmission of infectious disease, not to mention the fact that many people are simply uncomfortable with the idea.

Synthetic implants are nonhuman, nonanimal polymers that are placed permanently in the skin. *Polymers* are tiny molecules strung in long, repeating chains. Polymers such as the synthetic product Gore-Tex are commonly used to repair major blood vessels and in reconstructive plastic surgery. Polymers can be permanently implanted beneath deep acne scars. A problem with these polymer implants is that their bulk is easily felt when touching the skin. Some people find this unacceptable.

In this chapter, I've presented a large number of treatment options falling into many broad categories. You may be feeling somewhat overwhelmed by all of these possibilities. Any medical decisions should be made together with an appropriately trained and board certified medical professional. In the next chapter, I'll provide some general treatment recommendations and guide you in choosing the most effective treatment for your acne.

5

What Treatment Option Is Right for You?

Acne and its response to treatment is a function of your own specific physiology and personal preferences. What works well for your friend and seems to agree with her skin chemistry may not work for you at all. I frequently see despair in my new patients who tried their best friend's miraculous acne product, only to find that it caused a skin rash and made their acne worse. Acne is like many other things in life. For example, a low-fat, high-protein diet works well for some, while it is disastrous for others. It's all about how things interact with your specific chemistry. This is why blanket statements about what acne treatments are good for everyone are inevitably wrong.

You are learning throughout this book how to be a skilled observer of your skin. There is both the science of skin care and a trial-and-error component for each person. While I can make statistically sound generalizations about your skin type, they may or may not apply to you. Until medicine and science give dermatologists the tools to precisely assess your individual body chemistry, you must carefully observe your own skin reactions to treatments and change regimens as necessary. The Daily Acne Log (exercise 3.2) can help you to follow your specific skin reactions. Rest assured, it is always possible to find a treatment regimen that works well for you and your skin.

YOUR ACNE IS NOT A LOST CAUSE

A patient of mine once said, "I swam frantically for so long against the tide of acne, the thought of giving up, going with the tide, and hiding from life almost felt like a welcome relief." It is practically inevitable that if you have been suffering from ongoing acne, you feel to some degree like a lost cause. After all, everyone else need only use their over-the-counter or Internet miracle overnight acne cure, and you are barraged with images of their smiling faces and perfect skin. Why are you so different from them? What is wrong with you that makes you such a miserably resistant and hopeless case?

The answer to that question is that you are not different from the majority of acne sufferers. There are those lucky few who respond immediately to treatment or simply outgrow their pimples seemingly overnight. But for most people, acne is a stubborn skin condition that is often slow to respond. The images that are presented to you in magazines and on TV are simply not attainable by most in the real world. In reality, even the best of acne treatments take several weeks—if not longer—to yield any noticeable improvement.

I know that is not what you want to hear. You want your acne gone tonight, or tomorrow at the latest. Human nature is composed of very powerful basic survival instincts that are aroused when anything causes you pain or jeopardy, physical or emotional. Acne causes pain, sometimes both physical and emotional. Therefore, the anguish, desperate frustration, and anger that all acne sufferers sometimes feel is an inevitable manifestation of basic human nature. So of course you are drawn to and tempted by the miraculous promises made by these solicitors.

YOU CAN CONTROL YOUR ACNE

Now that you understand the basics of acne, you know that some people have stubborn pore cells that will continue to misbehave for much of their adult life. Therefore, for many people, cure is not possible. However, acne can virtually always be well controlled. Controlling your acne may be very simple, requiring only modest efforts and the use of over-the-counter products. However, if you are like most of the people I work with, the treatment equation will probably be a little more difficult. Good control may require prescription topical and oral medications alone or together with newer laser and other light therapies. Creative regimens are the specialty of dermatologists, and usually a treatment can be found to suit your specific needs. There are no lost causes or hopeless, pitiful creatures that defy all science. What I do frequently see are people who have become fatigued, disillusioned, and angry because of the numerous unsuccessful therapies that created a vicious cycle of enthusiasm and optimism that only led to feelings of defeat and despair.

The essence of what I am saying is this: Don't give up. There are so many new and emerging therapies that are safe and effective. Don't miss out.

GENERAL TREATMENT RECOMMENDATIONS

Knowing your skin type can help you choose a skincare regimen for acne. Dry skin generally responds better to treatment products formulated as creams or ointments, because they hydrate the skin. If you have oily skin, gels and lotions are usually preferable, since they can be drying and don't add oil to your skin.

Watch out for strong or allergic reactions to skincare products. Most acne products can be somewhat drying and irritating for some people. If you experience mild dryness or redness, I suggest that you decrease the frequency of application (for example, use it every other day rather than daily). Consider adding a moisturizer if your skin becomes too dry. Do not be concerned that moisturization will cause additional breakouts. As long as you gently cleanse the skin before application, moisturizers will not cause acne. Persistent or intense redness accompanied by itching or burning should alert you to the possibility of allergy or excessive irritation. You should always be vigilant for scars at the site of acne breakouts. If you observe any scarring, consult with a physician as soon as possible.

This section will provide you with specific treatment approaches for mild, moderate, and severe acne. This classification can serve as a reference to help guide you toward an appropriate treatment regimen.

Mild Acne

Mild acne consists of blackheads, whiteheads, small red bumps, or a combination of the three.

- Begin treatment with an over-the-counter wash, gel, or cream containing benzoyl peroxide, salicylic acid, or both (Oxy 5, Persagel, SalAc).

- Complete the Acne Trigger Identifier (exercise 3.1) to identify lifestyle or emotional factors that contribute to your acne.

- Consider glycolic acid washes or peels (available over the counter or in a dermatologist's office).

- Consider gentle facials with extraction.

- If your acne persists, try a prescription topical retinoid cream or gel (Retin-A, Differin, Tazorac, Velac).

- If acne persists, add a prescription antibiotic product such as benzoyl peroxide with clindamycin (BenzaClin, Duac), clindamycin (Clindagel, Clindamax, Cleocin), sodium sulfacetamide with or without sulfur (Klaron, Rosac, Rosanil, Rosula, Clenia), or niacinamide (Nicomide).

- If acne persists, seek a prescription for an oral antibiotic agent: low-dose doxycycline (Periostat), higher-dose doxycycline (Doryx, Adoxa), minocycline (Dynacin), or erythromycin (PCE, Eryc).

- If acne is still present, an oral contraceptive, spironolactone (Aldactone), or both may be helpful.

- If acne is still present, laser or photodynamic therapy may be effective.

- If acne is still present and causes scarring or extreme emotional impact, consider isotretinoin (Accutane, Sotret, Amnesteem, Claravis).

Moderate Acne

Moderate acne consists of blackheads, whiteheads, numerous raised (inflamed) red bumps, persistent cystic acne along the jawline, or a combination of these.

- Moderate acne needs medical evaluation. Until your medical appointment, use a topical product with benzoyl peroxide, salicylic acid, or both.

- Complete the Acne Trigger Identifier (exercise 3.1) to identify contributing lifestyle and emotional factors.

- You will probably need combined therapy: an oral antibiotic agent with a topical retinoid and a topical antibiotic combination.

- If acne persists, an oral contraceptive, spironolactone, or both may be helpful.

- If your acne is still present, laser or photodynamic therapy may be effective.

- If your acne is still present and causes scarring or extreme emotional distress, consider isotretinoin.

Severe Acne

Severe acne causes deep, painful cysts and obvious scarring.

- Acne that is severe needs prompt medical evaluation by a dermatologist. Topical therapy is usually of no substantial benefit.

- Complete the Acne Trigger Identifier (exercise 3.1) to identify lifestyle and emotional factors that may be contributing to your acne.

- You will almost definitely need oral antibiotic therapy.

- If your acne persists, an oral contraceptive, spirono-lactone, or both may be beneficial.

- If acne persists, laser or photodynamic therapy may be helpful.

- Oral isotretinoin may be necessary for adequate control.

Extremely resistant acne or acne that is leaving scars on the skin should be evaluated by a dermatologist. The dermatologist has the largest knowledge base and most complete array of therapies to improve your acne and your skin.

TRACKING THE EFFECTIVENESS OF TREATMENT

Fair and accurate assessment of the effectiveness of your acne treatment can be difficult. You certainly despise your pimples, and it often seems like an eternity before a breakout subsides and disappears. Because of this, many people simply jump ship, abandoning a treatment regimen before giving it a chance to work. Keep in mind that each new breakout that appears on your skin actually began forming about three weeks earlier. Therefore, even with the best of treatments, there is always a lag of at least three weeks before any obvious decrease in breakouts can be seen.

I encourage you to track the effectiveness of your treatment using the Acne Monitoring Chart (exercise 5.1). Make several copies of the blank chart so you will have a fresh copy each week. It should take you no more than about twenty seconds to complete the chart each morning. Quickly count the number of blackheads and whiteheads and the number of red bumps. If you are unsure, round off to the higher number. Keep the chart in the bathroom on the sink or in the medicine chest.

EXERCISE 5.1: ACNE MONITORING CHART

Monday begins week of month/day: _____

Current medications: _____

_____

Fill in the number of blackheads/whiteheads and red bumps for each day of the week. Since these last longer than a single day, you will be counting the same ones more than once. At the end of the week, add up the total number of blackheads/whiteheads for the week and the total number of red bumps.

	Blackheads/Whiteheads	Red Bumps
Monday		
Tuesday		
Wednesday		
Thursday		
Friday		
Saturday		
Sunday		
Totals:		

After approximately four to six weeks of effective acne treatment, your numbers should begin to decrease. If you don't see any improvement, consider adding to or changing your skincare regimen. Determining which aspect of the skincare regimen to change is not always easy. It can be helpful to continue keeping your Daily Acne Log (exercise 3.2). If you find that a product is overly irritating or unpleasant to use, consider using it less often, discontinuing it, or substituting a different product. Essential parts of your regimen—such as topical retinoids, benzoyl peroxide products, topical antibiotics, and oral antibiotics—should be changed only after consulting your skincare professional. Often, major changes in your regimen are not necessary to improve control of your acne. Changing your diet, better managing stress, or adding or substituting a medication is frequently all that is necessary.

6

The Psychological
Effects of Acne

Your acne and your emotions are inevitably linked. In this chapter, we'll take a look at how acne is related to your emotions. First, though, I'd like you to meet Brooke.

▪ Brooke

Brooke closed her eyes tightly, trying desperately to squeeze away the anxiety, fear, and sadness that had become her nighttime torture. She would usually wake up abruptly in a cold sweat after only a few hours of sleep, her heart racing and her body trembling. The relentless and overwhelming silence of the middle of the night only intensified her anxiety and near panic. Images of social ridicule and rejection rapidly flashed through her mind as she prayed for morning to come. She had felt sure that these terrible nights that had tormented her as a teenager were gone for good. Why now, why again? Was the recurrence of her "teenage acne" that now covered her face and back somehow related to her anxiety and depression? The answer is yes, but first I need to ask you to leave Brooke for the moment and come with me to my psychodermatologist psychotherapy couch.

ACNE AND SELF-IMAGE

Let's talk about your identity, your sense of who and what you are: what is colloquially called your self-image. Like every human being, you are a collection of inborn biological predispositions that are challenged and modified by your life experiences. Your interactions with parents, siblings, relatives, friends, teachers, bosses, coworkers, and even strangers affect you. Chance life experiences (who you sat next to in kindergarten, painful and embarrassing moments, early successes and failures), illnesses, injuries, and environmental exposures affect you as well. These numerous factors can strengthen and build or weaken and scar your private, inner sense of who you are.

Acne has a uniquely strong potential to leave not only physical but also emotional scars, since it is an extremely visible affliction associated with many myths about cleanliness, purity, self-control, intelligence, and diet. For some, acne represents only a small burden and challenge, while for others, it can be a devastating experience, the final straw in a difficult life. Acne combines with your other life experiences to determine your self-image and the manner in which you interact with others. Your internal emotional world, outgoingness, comfort in social situations, assertiveness, sensuality, and sexuality are all affected.

Let's get more specific now and talk about you and me. Close the door, lie back, and make sure that no one else is listening, because I want to share with you some secrets that I have learned from the thousands of acne patients I have treated. Some might call them dirty little secrets, because they apply to all of us, whether we admit to them or not. Take a deep breath, because here we go.

I know that despite that confident facade you wear in your work and social interactions, sometimes you are simply hiding—afraid or even terrified—behind that mask of social self-confidence. If it is any consolation, so am I. The truth is, most of us feel deep down that we are not attractive enough, not smart enough, not competent enough, and therefore live in fear of being exposed for who and what we really are. We look around us, and everyone else seems so self-confident and together, free of insecurities and self-doubts like ours. Guess what? What you see is not what you get. Those "perfect" people are just like you and me. The bottom line is that we all desperately seek and need the approval and acceptance of others, often to a pathological extent. Another secret is that everyone sometimes gets really scared in the middle of the night, often for no apparent reason.

Finally, in order to keep going and feel good inside, we all need a genuine, heartfelt hug and pat on the back on a regular basis. If you interact with children, you know that this is a no-brainer. The hungry look in their eyes, the desperate need for approval after performing a task, compels us to offer praise and affection. Our hugs and smiles are soaked up, filling that invisible reservoir of approval and acceptance that later supplies their self-confidence. So why must that end? Why are open expressions of praise, acceptance, and affection replaced with verbal expressions such as *not bad, adequate, could have been better?* School grades, performance evaluations, and sales quotas just don't satisfy the basic needs for approval and affection that persist throughout life.

These needs for acceptance and affection are utterly essential. Consider the concept of "failure to thrive." It was originally described during the World War II, when orphaned children, despite adequate nutrition, began to wither and die. Their conditions were reversed only when they were held and interacted with in a positive way (Spitz 1945). Similar observations have been made about elderly adults living alone (Robertson and Montagnini 2004). Children and adults must be touched and interacted with in order to survive. Those denied touch will wither and die, while those held and touched can flourish.

So what is the take-home message? Do not allow your acne to prevent you from experiencing life-sustaining and life-enriching touch. Touch need not be romantic or sexual; it can be the simple warmth of a handshake, the pleasant sensation of a gentle pat on the arm, or the delightful experience of receiving or giving a hug. Touch can also be felt in nonphysical ways. A smile or friendly voice can "touch" you and bring about those positive physiological changes. Opportunities are everywhere: with friends, with family, at work, in houses of worship, and in volunteer organizations—even at the corner coffee shop.

Most of us perceive ourselves as scarred, imperfect, flawed, and frightened human beings. Each of us is ignorant about many things and incompetent in many ways. I know more secrets about you: You can be a little nutty. You are sometimes moody, sometimes sad and miserable, sometimes anxious, often angry. The problem with acne is that it adds one more big, ever visible flaw to the list of flaws you believe yourself to have, and that list is already pretty long.

What a mess. How can you actually feel good and comfortable in this life? The answer is, you can, and it is largely independent of how perfect your skin, body, hair, nails, or clothes are. It is all in your head . . . really. Specifically, the answer is based in your interpretation of reality.

YOUR THOUGHTS DETERMINE YOUR FEELINGS

Perception is in the eyes of the beholder. Much of happiness is independent from actual life circumstance. It is your thoughts that largely determine your feelings, and I can prove it to you.

Imagine this situation. Three thirty-five-year-old women, all with a lot of acne on the face and chest, attend a holiday party. Each is told by the same person at the party, "I notice that you have some acne on your forehead." The first woman is quite pleased because she is relieved that the other acne lesions on her face, chest, and back were not noticed. The second woman is slightly insulted and upset, blushes a little, but returns her focus to the party and is able to enjoy herself. The third woman is devastated. She blushes visibly and begins to perspire. Tears fill her eyes as she runs from the party and immediately drives home. Feeling distraught, she considers quitting her job and even entertains thoughts of suicide.

The same event took place for each of these three women, but look how very different their emotional and physical responses were. The determining factor in how they reacted was not the actual event but rather what each woman told herself about the event. The first woman was not pleased by the comment but focused on the positive aspect that the rest of her acne was not noticed. Therefore, she had little negative emotional response. The second woman perceived the comment about her skin as unpleasant and embarrassing but not catastrophic. Thus she was able to modulate the intensity of the negative response and let it go. The third woman clearly perceived the comment as a catastrophic, horrible experience, and she had intensely negative emotional, physical, and cognitive (thought) reactions.

This is the basis of a school of psychotherapy called *cognitive behavioral therapy*. Simply stated, thoughts—not events—cause feelings. It is what you tell yourself about life events rather than the events themselves that determine how you feel. Sure, certain really bad events will inevitably make you feel sad. However, it is your perceptions and *self-talk* (what you tell yourself) about the events that determine the intensity and duration of your emotional and physical response. Many people believe their responses to life events are fixed, as though they are hardwired or etched in stone. Statements such as "That's just how I am" are shining examples of the deeply held belief that change is impossible. In fact, these perceptions or self-talk can be changed, and modifying them can change how you experience your day-to-day life.

Let me prove this point. Imagine that you have a mole on your cheek that you hate. Your self-talk about the mole runs along the lines of *It makes me unattractive and ugly*. As time goes on, you find yourself thinking *I can't stand that mole. I would give anything to not have to live with that stupid thing.* One day, a well-intentioned friend tells you that an acquaintance just died of malignant melanoma, and her melanoma looked exactly like your mole. You suddenly become terrified that this "ugly mole" is actually a cancer. Despite urgent phone calls, it takes three weeks until an appointment with a dermatologist can be arranged. Upon close inspection, the dermatologist assures you that the lesion is absolutely not cancerous and in fact is identical in appearance and location to the mole on Cindy Crawford's face. Moreover, he emphatically tells you that removal of the mole would leave a large, unsightly surgical scar. Immediately, you feel a flood of relief, and this previously unbearable mole suddenly stops eliciting negative feelings. It is not that the mole has changed; it is what you tell yourself about the mole that has changed.

So wherever you find yourself on the emotional spectrum of acne sufferers, happy and unaffected or tragically burdened and depressed, you can modify your thoughts and emotional responses if you desire. The ideal acne treatment involves not only effective treatment of the acne lesions but also examination—and, if necessary, modification—of your response to the acne. I'll offer specific tips and exercises in chapter 8.

PSYCHOLOGICAL CONDITIONS ASSOCIATED WITH ACNE

There are several psychological conditions that are more commonly seen in acne sufferers. Whether the condition preceded the acne or occurred as a result of living with acne is not always clear. In fact, I do not believe that it is necessary to solve this "which came first" puzzle. What is more important is to recognize these disorders and, if you think that you are suffering with one of them, seek appropriate treatment. Acne excoriée, obsessive-compulsive disorder, depression, anxiety, and body dysmorphic disorder are psychological conditions that are commonly seen in association with acne.

As you read about each of these disorders, you may experience the "I think that's me" syndrome frequently observed in students of psychology and psychiatry. It is common for medical students and mental health professionals in training to read the symptoms of psychiatric disorders and conclude with certainty that they suffer from each one of them. In other words, I expect you will find that you have some of the symptoms of these disorders. It is the extent to which these behaviors and thoughts interfere with your ability to be happy and to function effectively in life that determines whether you actually have the disorder and need treatment.

Acne Excoriée

Acne excoriée is a condition in which people with acne pick, scratch, or dig at their acne lesions. Most people with acne will manipulate their lesions from time to time, either squeezing them or picking at them. What distinguishes acne excoriée from the common manipulation of acne is the extent of the manipulation. People with acne excoriée pick, scratch, or dig at their skin to the extent that open sores and scabs are frequently visible. Even more distressing is the fact that many people with acne excoriée manipulate the skin to the point of scarring. The skin often becomes a sea of active sores, scabbed lesions, and scars from previous picking. Substantial hyperpigmentation (darkening of the skin in spots) may result from all the manipulation and inflammation. The sight of these skin alterations causes emotional distress that leads to more picking.

Some acne excoriée sufferers stop their skin manipulation once their acne has abated. Many times, however, acne excoriée takes on a life of its own, and the affected person continues to pick at the skin even in the absence of any active acne. If you have active acne and acne excoriée, both the acne and the picking must be treated. If you pick at your skin even though there is no active acne present, only the picking needs to be treated. Nonetheless, I recommend a therapeutic skin lotion such as glycolic acid or stabilized vitamin C acid together with a topical retinoid to promote skin health and resolution of hyperpigmentation.

In order to be effective, treatment of acne excoriée must take into account the fact that the urge to pick can be very powerful and compelling. High levels of internal tension and distress often accompany the urge or compulsion to pick. Simple admonishments by loved ones, such as "Don't pick" and "Stop picking," are almost universally useless. These statements tend to elicit frustration and anger that can actually lead to more picking. In order for you to pick less and eventually stop picking, two things are necessary: you need alternative behaviors, and you need methods to decrease internal tension and distress.

Having a menu of alternative behaviors can be enormously helpful. Without the option of an alternative behavior, when a strong urge to pick occurs, you can either pick or simply hope the urge will pass. Very simple alternative behaviors include doing finger exercises, squeezing a stress ball, or playing with worry beads. You can gently apply acne medications to your skin, being cautious not to overuse potentially irritating products that can cause skin rashes. Better yet, you can use a stress management technique (like deep breathing, guided imagery visualizations, or progressive muscle relaxation, each of which I'll teach in chapter 8) as an alternative behavior. These alternatives to picking will gradually become incorporated as your response to acne and stress and therefore replace your skin picking.

Sometimes, the compulsion to pick and the associated emotional discomfort require medication in addition to the above techniques. Antidepressant and antianxiety medications can be very effective in enhancing your ability to control unwanted behaviors and decrease emotional distress.

Obsessive-Compulsive Disorder

Obsessive-compulsive disorder (OCD) shares some features with acne excoriée. Like people with acne excoriée, OCD sufferers engage in compulsive behaviors. The urge to perform these behaviors is often accompanied by a substantial amount of emotional discomfort that is temporarily relieved by performance of the compulsive act. People with OCD engage in a wide array of compulsive acts, including manipulation of the skin. Other common compulsions are checking, washing, praying, or repeating words.

The other feature of OCD is obsessions. Obsessions are unwanted ideas or impulses that repeatedly well up in the mind of the person with OCD. Persistent fears that harm may come to you or a loved one, an unreasonable concern with becoming contaminated, or an excessive need to do things correctly or perfectly are common. Again and again, the person experiences a disturbing thought, such as *My hands may be contaminated—I must wash them, I may have left the gas on,* or *I am going to injure my child.* These thoughts are intrusive and unpleasant, and they produce a high degree of anxiety. Obsessive thoughts about acne or other skin imperfections are common. Sometimes the obsessions are of a violent or sexual nature, or they may center on concerns about illness.

Obsessive-compulsive disorder is best treated with a combination of antidepressant medication and behavioral psychotherapy. This combination has proven very effective in freeing OCD sufferers from the intrusive and troubling burden that these thoughts and impulses pose. If you fear that your obsessions and compulsions may cause you to harm yourself or others, you must seek immediate evaluation and treatment. Many people with OCD have troubling thoughts about behavior that is aggressive or otherwise unacceptable. Despite the occurrence of these thoughts, OCD rarely actually causes people to harm themselves or anyone else.

Body Dysmorphic Disorder

Body dysmorphic disorder (BDD) is a serious problem of impaired perception that may be related to obsessive-compulsive disorder. Those who have BDD are abnormally preoccupied with a real or imagined defect in their physical appearance. The skin, hair, and nose are the most common areas of preoccupation. For example, those affected with BDD may worry endlessly that their skin is pale, their hair is too curly, their nose is too long, or something else is wrong with the way they look. When others tell them they look fine or the flaw isn't noticeable, people with this disorder don't hear or believe it. The person with BDD may also experience periods of depression, anxiety, and even suicidal thoughts because of the preoccupation with the perceived flaw.

BDD is different from the distortions and dissatisfaction that all of us have with our skin and body. We all have a tendency to magnify and focus on those aspects of our appearance that we wish were different. According to Gupta and Gupta (2001a), 56 percent of the general population report dissatisfaction with the appearance of their skin. The key distinguishing factor of BDD is that sufferers have substantial impairments in their quality of life. The obsessive preoccupation can make them unable to work, socialize, and interact with family members. BDD sufferers are frequently unavailable to others due to long hours spent in front of a mirror. Most suffer from the belief that others are staring at them or talking about their imperfections.

Treatment of BDD must include both antidepressant medication and cognitive behavioral psychotherapy. Sometimes, low doses of psychiatric medications used for psychosis are necessary. Although the obsessive preoccupations are often not eliminated even with successful therapy, they can usually be reduced to manageable levels that interfere less with quality of life. If suicidal thoughts and impulses are present, immediate psychiatric attention is essential.

Depression and Anxiety

Anxiety and depression are prevalent in acne sufferers. This is hardly surprising, given that even in the absence of the disorders I've just discussed, one's appearance has a tremendous influence on self-image. Difficulties with self-image are intimately linked with anxiety and depression. In chapter 8, I'll help you determine whether anxiety and depression are interfering with your quality of life. Chapter 8 also includes many tools to help you cope with stress and reduce your symptoms of anxiety and depression.

RESEARCH ABOUT THE EMOTIONAL EFFECTS OF ACNE

I want to briefly review some of the data showing the powerful emotional impact acne can have. Remember, the severity of acne (how many pimples you have and how large or how red they are) does not necessarily predict how emotionally affected you will be.

Clinical depression, social phobia, anxiety disorders, and anger have been proven to be associated with acne. Unbelievable to all except people who suffer from acne, the studies show that these negative emotional reactions are greater in acne sufferers than in people with other medical problems, including cancer (Kellett and Gawkrodger 1999). Acne sufferers have a higher incidence of suicidal thoughts than people with other dermatological disorders (Gupta and Gupta 1998). Studies have shown that acne can cause impairment in self-image and self-esteem, impairment in overall psychological well-being, dissatisfaction with appearance, and problems with social interactions (Lasek and Chren 1998).

Another way in which the effects of acne are measured is looking at a person's quality of life. Quality of life measures assess whether a condition interferes with people's ability to engage in their usual range of life activities and their ability to experience pleasure in life. Many studies have confirmed that acne does indeed reduce quality of life. In fact, the impact is as great as that experienced by people suffering from chronic, disabling asthma, epilepsy, diabetes, and arthritis (Kellett and Gawkrodger 1999). Another study showed that adults with acne suffer even greater negative effects on quality of life than younger acne sufferers (Lasek and Chren 1998).

A recent study in the *British Journal of Dermatology* (Rapp, Brenes, and Feldman 2004) looked specifically at anger and acne and the implications for quality of life and patient satisfaction. Their findings suggested that anger among people with acne was more related to the emotional impact of acne than to the severity of the acne. Acne did, as expected, have a significant negative impact on reported quality of life. Chronic anger seemed to predispose people to react more negatively to skin disease. The study also found that social sensitivity was related to the degree of distress associated with acne. People with higher degrees of social sensitivity are more shy and worried about what others think of them. When their acne is worse, they are more distressed and potentially more prone to have worsening of their acne in response to their distress. A vicious cycle of distress and acne can evolve. Both anger and social sensitivity are personality traits that can be modified by many techniques, including progressive muscle relaxation, guided imagery, cognitive behavioral therapy, yoga, and tai chi.

Beyond the emotional impact, there is no doubt that acne can substantially interfere with functioning. Acne sufferers have decreased involvement in sports, eat out less, date less, and have poorer academic performance (Motley and Finlay 1989). People with acne were found to have significantly higher unemployment rates (16.2 percent versus 9.2 percent in a 1986 study by Cunliffe), underscoring the potential economic impact of acne.

EFFECTIVE ACNE TREATMENT CAN HELP RELIEVE ITS EMOTIONAL EFFECTS

There is, however, some really good news. Effective acne treatment can reverse many of the negative emotional effects of acne. Each day in my office, I have the privilege of watching and sharing in the return of happiness in my patients as their acne is better controlled. It often seems to me as though someone has lifted a hundred-pound knapsack off the patient's back. They sit more erect and stand taller in my exam room. No longer ashamed of their skin, they look me directly in the eyes and maintain eye contact as they speak, allowing for a true intellectual and emotional exchange. Quality of life clearly improves. Patients share with me their return to or entrance into a fuller range of social and recreational activities. They are no longer seeking the darkest spot in the room, avoiding pools and beaches, and hiding at home. They can wear normal cosmetics, and their choice of clothing is no longer governed by where the pimples are.

■ Brooke

What about Brooke, who you met at the beginning of this chapter? Brooke's nighttime misery and her extensive acne were definitely related. She noted that her current trouble with acne had started at almost exactly the same time as her anxiety and depression. Anxiety and depression, like acne, can be triggered by hormonal changes and, conversely, can cause hormonal changes. The stress of Brooke's acne clearly contributed to the anxiety and sadness that had become pervasive in her life, while the anxiety and sadness negatively influenced her hair follicles, thereby worsening her acne. The question of which came first, the acne or the anxiety and depression, was irrelevant, since both had to be addressed.

Her treatment consisted of low-dose doxycycline, a topical retinoid, a combination benzoyl peroxide– clindamycin gel, glycolic acid peels, topical stabilized vitamin C, topical green tea polyphenols, oral omega-3 supplementation, and biofeedback therapy. Her acne gradually cleared over a three-month period, and her anxiety and depression abated.

To sum things up, there exists a reciprocal reaction or two-way street. Acne can cause stress and negative emotions. Stress and negative emotions can cause and worsen acne. Therefore, effective acne treatment should address both the acne lesions and the emotional state of the person with those lesions. In chapter 8, I'll offer stress reduction exercises and techniques for relieving anxiety and depression. These tools can be invaluable in helping you improve your acne and your quality of life.

7

Exploring Your Psyche

This chapter is perhaps the most demanding and challenging of any in this book. I am going to ask you to engage in some meaningful intro-spection designed to help you better understand what is going on in your inner world. Your goal is to identify thoughts and perceptions that may be causing you stress and distress. Both stress and distress negatively affect the quality of your life and may be worsening your acne.

PAYING ATTENTION TO THE PSYCHE

Like most people, you probably go through the motions of your daily life giving little attention or thought to that ever active and profoundly important inner world, the psyche. The *psyche* is the total sum of the vast collection of inborn tendencies (the temperament) that is contin-ually modified by your life experiences, including memories, hopes, aspirations, disappointments, conflicts, self-appraisals, and impulses. You learn to filter, suppress, and ignore many of the messages from the inner psyche, since they can be intrusive, distracting, and at times dangerous to your daily appropriate behavior.

I am not suggesting that you should unleash all the components of your psyche. Rather, I am advocating an honest, introspective evaluation of your ongoing thoughts and perceptions and how they relate to your overall happiness. This essential self-assessment method can allow you to achieve more happiness by modifying your thoughts and perceptions. Honest introspection requires you to carefully examine your internal emotional responses and the thoughts and perceptions that precede or accompany them. This introspection will help you target areas of your life that are most associated with stress, distress, and unhappiness.

We all experience a wide range of emotions—sometimes many at once—as a normal part of the human experience. Anger, joy, jealousy, anguish, elation, anxiety, tranquillity, sadness, giddiness, fear, confidence, frustration, triumph, terror, and rage fill all of us at various times. An important question to examine is this: To what internal and external aspects of your existence are these emotions bound? I have found in my years of research and clinical practice that skin problems, including acne, can be intimately interwoven with powerful and often negative aspects of the psyche. Acne can be especially devastating to the psyche, since it so profoundly affects your perception of yourself and is literally always "in your face."

The question you should honestly answer is whether acne has had a significantly negative impact on your emotions and your life. If so, these negative effects can be modified and your life changed for the better. Your perspective on life and your emotional reactions are not hardwired like a computer. You need not be forced to respond in the same emotionally painful ways for a lifetime.

EXERCISE 7.1: THE STRESS-DISTRESS-UNHAPPINESS MONITOR

This tool will allow you to uncover thoughts and perceptions that cause or worsen your internal experience of stress, distress, and unhappiness. The thoughts and perceptions that accompany your feelings are a nearly silent and yet always present dialogue. The goal of this exercise is to develop a sophisticated listening device to amplify this ever present dialogue.

Most people are surprised to find that this dialogue is composed of strong and sometimes very judgmental statements. Words and phrases such as "should," "must," "awful," "terrible," "unfair," "insensitive," and "can't stand it" are common. Absolutes abound in our internal dialogues: *I could never be happy if my face wasn't clear*, or *He never listens*. "Never" is an absolute and probably an unfair exaggeration. I will talk more about this later, but now let's get down to business and crank up your listening device. I think you will be surprised at what you hear.

Over the next week, notice when you experience a negative emotion like the ones listed below. When this happens, take a moment to identify the feeling and the thoughts and perceptions you were having when the feeling began. Write down your observations below.

Feelings to notice: stressed, distressed, angry, furious, sad, anxious, tense, fearful, frightened, agitated, confused, overwhelmed, resentful, fragile, vulnerable, violated, abused, exploited, belittled, mocked, inadequate, foolish, stupid.

Feeling   **Thoughts and Perceptions**

The information that you have gleaned from this exercise presents an opportunity for meaningful change. You do not have to respond to your life with these thoughts and perceptions. They are yours to change if you so desire. The events and people that "make you feel that way" may not always be amenable to change, but your internal dialogue always is. In fact, it is not the events and people that "make you feel" as you do; it is your self-talk, that internal dialogue, that does. Now that you've identified the connections between your emotions and your thoughts and perceptions, when you get to chapter 8, you'll be ready to get to work and improve your life.

One caveat is the fact that sometimes feelings occur simply because they do. I believe that some internal feelings occur because of hormones, sugar levels, biorhythms, and random discharges of energy in the body. Therefore, there will be many times when you will not be able to tie a thought or perception to an emotion. Put another way, sometimes it is what it is. When this happens, your best bet is to accept the feeling for what it is and move on with your day until the feeling passes.

COPING WITH THE EFFECTS OF ACNE ON YOUR PSYCHE

In this chapter, you have identified some of the ways acne has caused you stress and unhappiness. Even though they are not necessarily part of your moment-to-moment consciousness, these thoughts and feelings are a constant presence and can affect your perceptions, your bodily reactions, and your skin. Now you can begin the process of improving the quality of your life. In this section, we'll look at how you can go about doing this.

Phantom Acne

You may have heard of phantom limb pain, a well-recognized phenomenon that occurs after limb amputation. Despite the absence of a hand, arm, foot, or leg, the affected person continues to experience sensations as if the limb were still there. Physicians believe that phantom limb pain is caused by imprinted memories and pathways in the brain that continue to be active as if the limb were still attached. These sensations are often very troubling to the affected people and serve as an ongoing reminder of their loss of a limb.

"Phantom acne" is my term for the persistent feelings of self-consciousness, unattractiveness, and even ugliness that continue to plague acne sufferers long after their active acne lesions have disappeared. Perhaps phantom acne, like phantom limb pain, is caused by imprinted memories and brain pathways. Years of upsetting reflections in the mirror and the associated negative perceptions of yourself can certainly etch deep emotional scars. Phantom acne is analogous to the way formerly overweight people continue to perceive themselves as heavy despite having attained ideal body weight.

I strongly believe that everyone suffers from phantom emotional intrusion from whatever difficult experiences they've overcome. If you have dealt with acne, you will always feel to some degree that your skin is flawed; this is a natural and expected outcome. Phantom acne becomes a major problem when there are gross distortions in your perceptions of your appearance, leading to substantial emotional distress or difficulties in functioning.

■ Lynn

Lynn is a classic example of a person suffering from phantom acne. She came to my office with very mild acne on her cheeks. Her lesions were easily camouflaged with a small amount of makeup. Soon after I asked her why she had come to see me, she burst into tears and shared with me that she felt hideously repulsive, to the point that she had entertained thoughts of suicide. She explained in detail how she would wear her hair in styles that would hide her face as much as possible. At work, she would keep her face turned downward toward her desk, avoiding eye contact with coworkers. Even when approaching the drive-through window at McDonald's, she avoided facing the security camera, fearing that her acne would be seen by the person taking her order.

Clearly, Lynn was suffering from phantom acne. In order to free herself from these crushing feelings of self-consciousness, Lynn had to learn to change her thoughts about herself and her appearance. Even if your acne lesions have responded to treatment, you may need to work to bring your thoughts and feelings in line with this new reality. Give yourself permission to be a person with mild acne or no acne. In the next chapter, I'll talk more about how changing your thoughts—including your thoughts about acne—can help you change your feelings about yourself. Lynn achieved her happiness with a combination of microdermabrasion and antidepressant medication. She now looks Ronald directly in the eyes at the McDonald's drive-through.

Avoiding Obsession

Alcoholics Anonymous has a wonderful expression to explain how people prone to alcohol abuse find themselves in trouble: "Any thought nurtured long enough becomes an obsession." This is a profoundly insightful and important observation. The more time, attention, and energy you give to a thought, the more compelling and powerful the thought becomes.

For example, imagine that it is 4:00 p.m. and you have had nothing to eat all day. Your stomach feels extremely uncomfortable and is rumbling frequently. Aware that you will be unable to eat for another hour, you find that thoughts of your favorite foods keep pushing their way into your consciousness, only worsening your intense sensations of hunger. Gradually, you are becoming obsessed with food, feeling as though you cannot wait one more minute to soothe your overwhelming hunger pangs.

Suddenly, the phone rings. You answer the phone and are immediately told that you have won $100,000 in a contest you entered several months ago. Feeling giddy and euphoric, you call everyone you know. Your mind is filled with images of white sand and turquoise blue water; a lavish Caribbean vacation surely awaits you. Well, what about your hunger? You forgot it completely in your excitement.

And so it goes for acne. Thoughts about acne can also be nurtured until they achieve the status of obsession. Endless hours can be spent lamenting your unfair affliction. Each acne lesion can be studied, palpated, manipulated, and treated again and again with topical medications. Long periods can be spent in front of the mirror. I urge you, do not give your life away to obsession. Each moment spent obsessing about acne is a precious moment that could be spent living.

Maybe you will receive that phone call telling you you've won $100,000. Better still, maybe you will make a phone call that leads to something even better than fleeting giddiness: friendship, love, and a meaningful existence.

Avoiding the Misery Response

Many of your responses to people and events in your life are conditioned responses. For example, perhaps you can remember being infatuated with someone at some point in your life. Let's say for illustration purposes that the name of that special someone was Jack. Now, before you met Jack, that name probably didn't elicit any particularly strong emotional response. However, once you met Jack and experienced whatever interaction led to the infatuation, someone needed only mention his name and substantial internal happenings took place. The thoughts of his smile, mysterious deep blue eyes, broad chest, and strong arms caused butterflies in your stomach, extra beats of your heart, and those warm, tingly sensations. These reactions became associated with your thoughts and experiences of Jack. This *conditioned response* is a prime example of how your thoughts, emotions, and physiology can be affected positively by life experience.

Now let's examine how your conditioned responses can go awry. Suppose things with Jack have taken a substantial turn for the worse. The bright smile and warm, mysterious eyes have been replaced by harsh grimaces, angry words, disinterest, or even abuse. Now, the name "Jack" elicits sadness, anger, confusion, and misery. Self-deprecating thoughts like *I'm not good enough, pretty enough, sexy enough, funny enough* permeate your thoughts. Nausea, stomachaches, headaches, and total loss of energy may accompany those miserable emotions. The same person has become associated with totally different emotional reactions, physical reactions, and thoughts.

Now ask yourself what emotional reactions, physical reactions, and thoughts have become conditioned responses associated with your acne. My guess is that sadness, anger, fear, anxiety, frustration, confusion, and disillusionment are but a few of the emotions you have experienced. Headaches, stomachaches, nausea, muscle pain, fatigue, and lethargy—as well as unpleasant skin sensations such as itching, burning, extreme sensitivity, pain, and crawling sensations—all have been reported as occurring in response to acne. Acne often elicits an unending litany of self-deprecating thoughts. The good news is that conditioned responses—including those about acne—can be modified. In chapter 8, I'll offer tools and techniques to help you do this.

WHAT REALLY MATTERS: COMMITTING TO A VALUED LIFE

Everyone should almost die, at least once, maybe even on a periodic basis. I know, now you think I've really lost it. Perhaps, but please read on. Imagine having a near-death scare like narrowly avoiding a fatal accident. Imagine leaving a restaurant moments before a raging fire consumes the building. What if you were diagnosed with a terminal illness, only to find out several days later that a mistake had been made and you were not sick at all?

This type of life experience can bring sudden lucidity to an otherwise cluttered and tormented mind. Put another way, the really good thing about almost dying is that it provides an opportunity for phenomenal mental clarity and life perspective. The pus bump, acne scar, few extra pounds, varicose veins, dirty kitchen floor, and your kids' sloppiness suddenly seem totally insignificant. Flowers, trees, sunsets, and loved ones miraculously achieve magnificence. The relief of being alive and having been granted a second chance can liberate a sea of emotions. Happiness and relief flood the body, leading to almost giddy exhilaration.

You really don't need to have a near-death experience. You do, however, need to make a commitment to pursuing a life with value and meaning. You have the opportunity each morning to view life as a gift given to you each and every day. If you choose to view your life as a gift, you are free to embrace it fully. Each day is filled with opportunities to see, taste, feel, and join in new activities. In contrast, if you take life for granted, misery is more likely to fill your world, compelling you to withdraw from life and all the wonders it can offer.

Your initial reaction may be *Okay, I'm glad that I am not maimed or dead, but my life is too difficult to be filled with happiness*. Well, an astonishing fact is that happiness is, to a large degree, independent of life circumstance (Cowley 2002). Unless you're facing extreme tragedy or starvation, you have a choice in your life. You can choose to focus on the positive and wonderful things in the world, or you can choose to focus on the negative. Each moment of every day is an opportunity to form new positive and healthful conditioned responses that can heal the skin and soul.

Now is the time for you to examine what are the important things in your life, the things that you truly value. Is it your family, your friends, your dog or cat, the people in your house of worship, your job and coworkers? Perhaps it is your outdoor garden, houseplants, knitting skills, musical talent, artistic ability, mechanical ability, or decorating skills. Maybe it is your honesty, sense of humor, creativity, integrity, loyalty, or work ethic.

Redefining what is of real meaning and value in your life can dramatically change your cognitive, emotional, and physiological reactions for the better. Examples and exercises in chapter 8 will start you on the road to change. If you find that practicing and embracing these techniques improves your life to the point that you feel satisfied, that is terrific. If the degree of change is less than you had hoped, or if stress, anxiety, and sadness are prominent parts of your life, then you may consider seeking out a skilled therapist. There are entire schools of psychology that have been developed to help people change their perceptions and thinking habits. This is challenging but very important work. Please don't feel discouraged. If change were easy, therapists wouldn't have jobs.

8

Coping with Stress, Anxiety, and Depression

Stress, anxiety, and depression are inevitable events in the course of human experience. Regardless of the external events that fill your present life, I am sure that you frequently feel stressed, anxious, sad, irritable, and even depressed. I specifically say "regardless of the external events" because sometimes, you feel your worst when your outside world is at its best. The reasons for this seemingly illogical fact are many, but hormonal fluctuations and alterations in brain chemistry probably are at the root of many of these unpleasant emotions. In addition, there is an ongoing internal dialogue appraising yourself and your life, and this dialogue, although often out of your awareness, significantly affects your emotional life.

Sustaining your psychological equilibrium and overall happiness through these ups and downs is akin to a roller-coaster ride. Some people are better than others at riding this roller coaster of life. The better riders realize that the downs are eventually followed by the ups. Even if you say that much of your life has consisted of downturns, the reality is that for almost everyone, there will be upturns in the future. Even more important is the fact that you can begin to plan and construct your own roller-coaster tracks and lessen the extremes of this emotional roller coaster of life. You can learn to better deal with stress, anxiety, and depression. These efforts will lead to less turmoil, more happiness, and probably better skin.

WHAT IS STRESS?

Stress is the wear and tear your body experiences as a result of what life brings and how you deal with it. Stress has physical and emotional effects on you and can create positive or negative feelings. Stress can be a positive influence, giving you energy and helping to push you to action and improved performance. As a negative influence, stress can create feelings of distrust, rejection, anger, and depression, all of which can lead to health problems such as acne, headaches, upset stomach, rashes, insomnia, ulcers, high blood pressure, heart disease, and stroke. Stress can either help you or hinder you, depending on how you react to it.

Anxiety and depression are common reactions to the stresses of life. How you react to stress will determine how much anxiety or depression you experience.

HOW DO YOU KNOW IF YOU ARE STRESSED, ANXIOUS, OR DEPRESSED?

Are you stressed, anxious, or depressed? My guess is that your initial response is *Of course I am. Isn't everyone who lives in this crazy world?* "Stressed out," "nervous wreck," and "totally depressed" are only a few of the expressions that have become part of the vernacular of our culture. These frequent references reflect a societal awareness that these are unpleasant emotional reactions that can have negative effects on how we feel and function. The actual internal experience that defines these emotional states varies from person to person. For some, stress and anxiety are merely mild feelings of tension and jitteriness;

however, for others, the experience can be much more dramatic and even devastating.

J.V., a longtime acne sufferer, told me that when she is very stressed, "It's like a boa constrictor encircling my chest. As the sensation squeezes tighter, the feelings of panic and desperation overcome me. I want to scream, I want to run, but I am too terrified and paralyzed to move." The intensity of the real physiological components of her stress is very clear. That can't be good for the body and the skin.

Now, let's take a closer and more personal look at how you are reacting to the stress in your life.

EXERCISE 8.1: ARE YOU EXPERIENCING STRESS, ANXIETY, OR DEPRESSION?

Check off each of the feelings and physical reactions that you commonly experience.

ANXIETY

- ☐ feelings of anxiety

- ☐ agitation

- ☐ irritability

- ☐ confusion

- ☐ nervousness

- ☐ frightening dreams

- ☐ decreased interest in sex or other pleasurable activities

- ☐ increased use of alcohol, drugs, or tobacco

- ☐ excessive energy or extreme lethargy

- ☐ persistent, repetitive thoughts

- ☐ headaches

- ☐ tense or painful muscles

- ☐ decreased energy

☐   gastrointestinal upset

☐   change in appetite

☐   change in bowel habits

☐   dizziness

☐   clenching jaw, grinding teeth

☐   light-headedness

☐   frequent sweating

☐   sleep impairment

DEPRESSION

☐   difficulty concentrating

☐   feelings of depression

☐   sleep impairment

☐   persistent negative thoughts

☐   feelings of worthlessness and poor self-esteem

☐   excessive fatigue

☐   change in appetite

☐   loss of interest in sex and other pleasurable activities

☐   pessimism

If you checked off one or many of the above, you have only proven that you are a living, thinking, feeling human being, not necessarily that you are overly stressed or depressed. We all experience many of these symptoms as part of living. However, if you experience some or many of these symptoms frequently or intensely, you are probably experiencing clinically meaningful amounts of anxiety or depression in response to your stress. Each of these can erode your quality of life and negatively affect your skin.

GENERAL RECOMMENDATIONS FOR BETTER STRESS MANAGEMENT

Identifying the important and unrelieved stressors in your life and becoming aware of their effect on you is an important start. However, recognition alone is not sufficient for reducing the harmful effects of stress. Just as there are many sources of stress, there are many possibilities for its management. However, all require work toward change: changing the source of stress or changing your reaction to it. How do you proceed?

In this section, I'll outline some general approaches to managing stress. Later in this chapter, I'll discuss more specific tools and techniques to help you achieve this goal.

Become aware of your stressors and your emotional and physical reactions to them. Take notice of your internal distress. Don't ignore it. Don't minimize and gloss over your problems. Determine what events in your life distress you. Listen carefully to your internal dialogue. What are you telling yourself about the meaning of these events? Assess how your body responds to specific stressors. Do you become anxious or physically upset? If so, in what specific ways? Refer to the list of symptoms in exercise 8.1.

Recognize that change is possible. Could you change your stressors by avoiding them or eliminating them completely? Is it possible to reduce the frequency of the stressors (spread out your exposures over a period of time instead of experiencing them daily or weekly)? Is it possible to shorten your exposure to stress, perhaps by taking a break or leaving the physical premises? Can you approach the stressor with a different goal or strategy? For example, you could aim to complete only half the task during a shorter exposure rather than trying to finish 100 percent of it. Or, you could decide that your goal is to complete your task, not to make your boss happy.

Reduce the intensity of your emotional reactions to stressors. Internal stress reactions are triggered by your perception of danger, physical or emotional. Are you viewing your stressors in exaggerated terms or taking a difficult situation and making it catastrophic? Are you setting the unattainable goal of pleasing everyone? Are you overreacting and viewing things as absolutely critical, with life-and-death urgency? Do you feel you must always prevail in every situation? Work at adopting more realistic and moderate views. Try to see the stress as something you can manage and deal with rather than something that overwhelms and overpowers you. Try to temper your extreme emotions. Put the situation in perspective. Do not labor on the negative aspects. Avoid the *What if . . .* , *It would be awful if . . .* , and *I couldn't stand it if . . .* type of self-talk.

Learn to moderate your physical reactions to stress. Slow, deep breathing will bring your heart rate and respiration back to normal. Relaxation techniques can reduce muscle tension. Biofeedback training can help you gain voluntary control over such things as muscle tension, heart rate, and blood pressure. Medications, when prescribed by a physician, can help in the short term in moderating your physical reactions. However, they alone are not the answer. Learning to moderate these reactions on your own is a preferable long-term solution.

Heal and build your physical reserves. Exercise three to four times a week for cardiovascular fitness. Moderate, prolonged rhythmic exercise—such as walking, swimming, cycling, or jogging—is best. Eat well-balanced, nutritious meals. Maintain your ideal weight. Avoid nicotine, excessive caffeine, and other stimulants. Mix leisure with work. Take breaks and get away when you can. Get enough sleep. Be as consistent with your sleep schedule as possible.

Maintain your emotional reserves. Develop some mutually supportive relationships. Pursue realistic goals that are meaningful to you, rather than goals others have for you that you do not share. Expect some frustrations, failures, and sorrows. Always be kind and gentle with yourself—be a friend to yourself.

THE STRESS CASCADE

The stress cascade begins when you interpret a life event as stressful. This interpretation occurs in the cortex of the brain. The cortex sends stress messages to the pituitary gland, which in turn sends its stress messages to the thyroid gland. The thyroid gland continues the cascade by releasing its stress hormones, which directly affect the adrenal glands and the testes or ovaries. Then, the adrenal glands and the testes or ovaries release hormones that directly affect the skin, causing pro-acne changes in the hair follicles and inflammation in the skin. Stress management techniques can interrupt this cascade at its origins in the brain, preventing the cascade of negative effects that ends with acne.

STRESS REDUCTION EXERCISES

You are probably experiencing a fair amount of healthy skepticism regarding your ability or perhaps even your desire to learn stress reduction techniques. After all, you may perceive yourself as a strong, thinking person or maybe as someone who is not very good at learning new things. Even worse, you may feel that you are a very stressed and uptight person, not the sort who can simply change who you are. Well, I have met hundreds of people in my professional life who have started our relationship with statements such as "This is just the way I am" or "There are certain things that just can't be changed." I am glad to say that these statements simply aren't true. These types of statements are, however, excuses for not trying, and they are genuinely believed by the people who espouse them. Let's see if I can convince you how easily certain emotional reactions are learned and how they can be unlearned. Stress management techniques are simply methods by which you can replace negative and potentially harmful physical and emotional reactions with more positive and healthful ones.

■ Brian

Brian came to see me two years ago with worsening acne and an embarrassing tendency to blush intensely when he was angry, stressed, or embarrassed. He told me that as a child, he would blush easily when embarrassed, but he seemed to outgrow this tendency during his teenage years. Now, at age thirty-eight, the blushing had returned in full force, accompanied by inflamed and tender acne lesions. Internally, Brian would often feel angry and stressed, and he frequently experienced a rapid heartbeat, tightness in the throat, jaw tension, and sweaty palms. He was distressed both by his outside symptoms of acne and blushing and by his uncomfortable emotional and physiological symptoms. When I suggested that modifying some of his internal emotional and physiological reactions might help both his skin and his quality of life, Brian simply laughed and said, "It's hardwired in me from the factory."

My response to Brian was one of feigned amazement. I told him that I had never met someone capable of being embarrassed, frustrated by traffic, angry with his wife, and ashamed of his lack of monetary success all at the moment of birth. After his annoyance at my sarcasm passed, we began to talk about how his negative emotional and physiological reactions were learned and became connected to people, places, and things. He told me he felt almost as if he were a puppet who helplessly went through the day as the puppeteer pulled his strings. My question to Brian was this: Why shouldn't he be able to learn to attach the strings to different emotions and physical reactions? Stress management is simply training the body to respond in a healthier and more positive way.

Brian, a former high school and college athlete, went on to embrace stress management techniques with the same fervor and enthusiasm he exhibited for his athletics. Each time we met, he shared with pride his triumphs over the seemingly small events in his life. His anger and blushing were replaced by mild annoyance and sometimes even humor. His acne, which had previously been unresponsive to doxycycline and Tazorac, was now almost completely clear. At the conclusion of our last meeting, Brian sought his revenge. Halfway out the door, he looked at me and said, "You see, it's about learning not to react to the small stuff. I don't know what you're talking about with that stuff about being hardwired from the factory." He smiled and softly closed the door.

There is one very important caveat that anyone suffering from stress must consider. There is always the possibility that a medical problem may be contributing to your symptoms. If you experience substantial physiological and emotional symptoms of stress, I urge you to visit your primary care physician to be evaluated for any correctable biological causes. For example, an overactive thyroid gland or mitral valve prolapse can cause symptoms that are similar to stress and anxiety. These conditions can usually be easily ruled out, allowing you to comfortably embrace stress management techniques.

The Relaxation Response

The *relaxation response* refers to a phenomenon described by Herbert Benson. The basis of the relaxation response is the reality that your body can be taught or conditioned to relax. Therefore, your bodily state at any given moment is not a fixed response that is out of your control. Negative physiological responses need not run amok, poisoning your mind and body with unhealthy thoughts and stress-related chemicals. These seemingly automatic responses are absolutely modifiable and can be brought under your voluntary control. They can be replaced by healthier thoughts, feelings, and physiological reactions that can make you a happier, healthier, and probably less acne-burdened person.

In *The Relaxation Response* (2000), Benson describes how the body can be conditioned or trained to achieve a more relaxed state. Benson's relaxation response, like many other forms of relaxation training and stress management, results in bodily responses that are healthier and physiologically more comfortable. When the body is in a state of relaxation, blood pressure and heart rate are normalized, the release of stress hormones and inflammatory chemicals is decreased, blood sugar is better controlled, pain is reduced, thoughts are clearer, and the emotional state is generally better.

I urge you to practice at least one stress management technique from this chapter daily. Relaxation training and stress management exercises are skills that virtually everyone can learn. They are skills that improve with practice; the more you practice, the more efficient and effective you become at positively modifying your physiological reactions.

Progressive Muscle Relaxation

Progressive muscle relaxation is a commonly taught and easily learned method of achieving tension reduction and relaxation. This technique reduces your overall level of muscle and emotional tension and can be a helpful part of your overall stress management program. Progressive muscle relaxation heightens your awareness of how stress leads to muscle tension and discomfort. Tense muscles create discomfort and distress, and this can lead to additional stress. A vicious cycle can evolve in which stress begets physical discomfort, leading to more stress. The stressed body often produces a wide array of stress hormones that can lead to inflammation, fatigue, and a diminished quality of life.

Anyone can learn progressive muscle relaxation. There are no good or bad students, and the technique is safe for people of all ages and people with all medical conditions. The fundamentals of progressive muscle relaxation are based on several proven assumptions:

- Muscle tension causes physical and emotional discomfort.

- Keeping muscles tense uses a great deal of vital bodily energy, leaving less available for other activities of daily living.

- Many people are unaware of their tense musculature and the associated discomfort.

- Even with awareness, most people assume that these muscles cannot be voluntarily relaxed.

- Voluntary control over muscle tension can be achieved with simple exercises that reduce tension and discomfort.

EXERCISE 8.2:
PROGRESSIVE MUSCLE RELAXATION

I recommend that you practice progressive muscle relaxation in a comfortable chair or lying on a bed, couch, or floor. Begin by sitting or lying quietly with your eyes gently closed and taking a brief internal inventory of any physical or emotional discomfort. For example, take mental note of a tension headache, stiff neck, or jittery stomach.

Now, we will begin a series of exercises in which you will be asked to tighten and then relax different muscle groups on your face, neck, arms, back, and legs.

Close your eyes as tightly as you can. Keep them squeezed shut for five seconds, and then allow them to relax. Take note of the discomfort associated with sustained contraction of the muscles around your eyes and contrast that discomfort to the relief you feel as the muscles are allowed to relax. With your eyes still gently closed, repeat this two times.

Now, focus on your jaw and cheeks. Bite down with your back teeth and feel the muscles in the cheeks and around the jaw tense up. Hold them tense for five seconds, and then release. As before, focus on the discomfort produced by the tense muscles and contrast that sensation to the release that occurs as you allow the muscles to relax. Again, repeat this two more times.

Now, let's focus on the forehead muscles. Tighten the forehead muscles as much as possible, making an angry and worried expression. Hold them tight for five seconds, and then release. Repeat this two more times.

Now, let's move to the muscles of the upper forehead and the scalp. Try moving your eyebrows upward and tensing the upper forehead muscles, keeping them tense for five seconds. Allow them to relax, and then repeat two additional times.

Moving now to the neck and upper back muscles, simultaneously pull up your shoulders and tilt your head back while pushing your upper arms and elbows straight back. The muscles in your neck and upper back should feel very tight. Hold them tight for five seconds, and then allow them to relax. Repeat this two more times, again taking note of the pleasant sensation as the tension leaves the muscles.

Next, tighten the muscles of your abdomen by making your belly as hard as possible, as if you were trying to stop a punch from knocking the wind out of you. Hold them tight for five seconds, then release. Repeat twice, noticing the sense of release as the muscles relax.

Next, make a fist and hold it tight for five seconds. Release the tension and allow the muscles to relax for a few seconds. Repeat this two more times. Now, tighten the muscles of the upper arm by curling up your forearm as if to show off your biceps. Hold them tight for five seconds, and then release. Repeat this two more times.

Next, work on the muscles in the buttocks and lower back by tightening and releasing them, five seconds each time. Finally, work on the muscles of the lower legs by fully extending your legs and pushing your heels out while simultaneously flexing your toes back toward your knees as far as you can. Allow yourself to feel the tightness and tension in your calves for five seconds, and then allow them to fully relax. Note how the discomfort disappears as the muscles relax.

Now, sit or lie quietly for several minutes, focusing on all of the muscle groups you have worked on. They are now much more relaxed. Allow yourself to experience the pleasant sensations that accompany this relaxation. In this more relaxed state, the muscles are using very little of your body's energy compared to the substantial amount that was needed to keep them tense and tight. Notice the wonderful feelings of relaxation and warmth that occur when tension and discomfort are released.

A critical element of progressive muscle relaxation is focusing on the mild discomfort associated with each muscle contraction. Contrast this discomfort to the pleasant sensations of relief and relaxation that occur as you release the tension from each muscle group. Each time you practice, you will become more attuned to the amount of tension in your muscles, and you will find that you can easily reduce the level of tension by tensing and relaxing the muscle group. You will notice that as a result of your practice, your ability to monitor and modify muscle tension during the course of your day will be enhanced. Even better, you will be able to easily reduce muscle tension quickly and inconspicuously by gently contracting and relaxing any tense muscles.

The benefits of practicing progressive muscle relaxation are far beyond simply learning to relax your muscles. You will actually make positive changes in your physiology that have been shown to improve your overall health while simultaneously boosting your sense of well-being.

Guided Imagery

Guided imagery is a useful and fun technique with proven effectiveness in medicine, business, performing arts, and sports. Using specific visualization techniques, you can learn to modify your attitudes, emotions, physiology, and performance. These modifications can help you decrease negative thoughts and the unpleasant emotional and physiological reactions that often accompany negative thoughts. You can build a more positive outlook on your life and your skin. The visualization exercises are designed to help you very specifically imagine yourself behaving and responding in the manner you wish. Guided imagery is also a method by which a therapeutic relaxation response can be achieved.

I am going to lead you through a guided imagery relaxation exercise designed especially for you as an acne sufferer. There are several goals of this exercise. The first goal is to make you feel more relaxed and more comfortable living in your skin, regardless of how perfect or flawed it is. The second goal is to positively influence your physiology, thereby optimizing your overall health. The third goal is to improve your skin chemistry by reducing the release of *neuropeptides* (proinflammatory chemicals released in the skin) and other inflammatory acne-producing and acne-worsening chemicals. In short, the global goal is to make you feel and look better. I have used guided imagery techniques in my clinical practice for more than twenty years. I find that guided imagery can be a powerful and liberating tool for improving acne and other common skin conditions. You may wish to make a recording of yourself (or someone else whose voice you find soothing) reading these instructions. A similar guided imagery exercise using my voice is available at yardleyderm.com.

EXERCISE 8.3: GUIDED IMAGERY

Now, let's begin. Find a place where you can sit comfortably, recline, or lie down. Ideally, this should be a time and a place where you are unlikely to be interrupted. If you are interrupted by the sound of a person's voice or the telephone, simply deal with the intrusion and then return to your imagery exercise.

Close your eyes, allowing your eyelids to rest without effort or tension. Focus only on your breathing for the next several moments. Take note of the slight effort required as you draw air into your lungs through your nose and mouth. Notice the pleasant feeling of fullness in your chest as your lungs fill with the wonderful and life-sustaining air. Now, as you exhale, take note of the effortless nature of exhalation and the pleasant sense of release that accompanies it. Allow your breaths to become slightly deeper and just a little slower than usual as you pay attention to the wonderful, rhythmic cycle of your body-enriching inhalations followed by the gentle and soothing exhalations. As you focus on this cycle of healthy breathing, you can actually feel yourself settling comfortably into the cushions or mattress upon which you are resting. As you continue your rhythmic breathing, I would like you to take a brief bodily inventory focusing on any areas of stress, muscle tension, skin eruptions, or pain. Make a brief mental note of these areas and then return your focus to your breathing.

Now, I would like you to take a very deep breath and hold it for approximately five seconds, then allow it to flow freely, without any effort, from your nose and mouth. Notice the sense of stretching and even discomfort as your lungs fill to near capacity, followed by the wonderful sense of release and relief as you allow the air to escape freely. Repeat this one more time, and this time, as you exhale, you can actually imagine your bodily tension, distress, and any pain being released from your body. Very good. Now return to your slow and rhythmic breathing and allow yourself to feel even more relaxed and more at ease.

Emerging from within you, in a subtle and reassuring fashion, is an inner sense of calm, control, and optimism. It is best described as a feeling of ability . . . an ability that enables you to better control your emotions and physiology. It is an ability that allows you to make changes and choices that are beneficial for your life and your skin.

Now, imagine looking in the mirror and seeing your acne or other imperfections. Rather than responding with negative thoughts and unpleasant inner sensations, focus on your eyes and ask yourself whether you wish to allow physical imperfections to own your emotions and happiness. I want you to take a deep breath, then begin the process of taking control. Imagine medicating your acne lesions, gently touching the skin with an over-the-counter spot gel or prescription medication. You may actually feel a tingling sensation in the skin as you imagine the medication clearing the skin of P. acnes and sweeping away any inflammatory cells. Imagine the acne lesions shrinking as if they were small puddles of water evaporating in the warm sun. You can feel a gentle sensation of warmth on the face, neck, back, chest, and arms. Your negative feelings about your acne seem less troubling, replaced by warm, relaxed, and positive sensations.

As you briefly visit the other areas of concern on your body or in your life, you feel an ability to choose how much of your time and energy they deserve. You can choose to hear a safe and soothing voice saying, "Let it go." You are the one with the ability to let go of troubling and intrusive thoughts, images, and feelings. Looking again in the mirror, you think quietly to yourself, I don't always like what I see, but I refuse to allow it to hurt me.

Returning now to your breathing, focus again on the air filling your lungs, followed by the pleasant release as you exhale. Allow your body to drift comfortably into your chair, couch, or bed and feel and enjoy a few more peaceful moments of relaxation.

Slowly now, begin to focus on your surroundings and allow these warm feelings to stay with you. You will keep with you all the feelings of control, optimism, and choice that you have released within yourself. You have the ability to bring back these feelings at any time you choose throughout the day. Simply take a deep breath, hold it, and then release it. This will become a familiar signal to your body that will reproduce the relaxation response, modify your reactions, and lead to the release of healthful chemicals in the body. You now have the ability to maintain your attitudes and physiology in a way that is healthful for body and skin.

Regular practice of this guided imagery exercise will yield ongoing benefits. You may choose to do this during the day, or you may do it as a means to relax and decompress immediately before sleep. Do not measure the success of your guided imagery training by the clarity of your skin. Improved mood, decreased inner tension and anxiety, and overall improvements in your day-to-day life are the true measures of success.

Yoga and Tai Chi

Yoga and tai chi are structured programs that have a long, proven history of reducing stress, improving mood and focus, and enhancing strength and flexibility. Many of my patients find that practicing yoga or tai chi enhances their overall feelings of well-being and improves their ability to deal with the stresses of everyday life. Yoga and tai chi can be learned and practiced at home using videotapes or DVDs. Most people report greater benefit from attending structured classes. These classes are widely available at schools, community centers, and fitness clubs.

Aerobic Exercise

It seems that aerobic exercise can benefit sufferers of virtually every malady that burdens humankind. *Aerobic exercise* is any activity that significantly elevates your heart rate for the duration of the activity. Stress, depression, anxiety, fatigue, arthritis, irritable bowel syndrome, headaches, pain syndromes, and heart disease all can be improved by exercise. Exercise also appears to have protective effects on the brain, decreasing your chances of developing Alzheimer's disease.

Since aerobic exercise has been proven to reduce stress and inflammation, it makes scientific sense that it should be beneficial for inflammatory skin conditions such as acne. However, I am not aware of any well-controlled study that has convincingly addressed this issue. In fact, some acne sufferers report that the perspiration and friction associated with exercising can worsen their acne. However, you can usually eliminate most of these exacerbating effects by wearing loose-fitting clothing and cleansing soon after exercising using an antibacterial wash containing benzoyl peroxide or salicylic acid.

Biofeedback Training

Biofeedback training has been used extensively in medicine and psychology for many years. It is a totally noninvasive technique that provides very specific feedback about your physiology. Typically, muscle tension is measured in millivolts by gentle sensor pads that sit atop the skin. Blood flow to your extremities is measured in degrees by a temperature probe that is taped or clipped to a finger or toe. More elaborate biofeedback monitors are available that can measure skin electrical conductivity (*galvanic skin response*) and brain activity (*electroencephalogram—EEG*). The basic tenet of biofeedback training is that by using the information provided to you by means of the sensors, you can learn to better recognize and voluntarily control your bodily reactions.

Like most people, you learned early on in life that there are certain aspects of your physiology that you can control and certain aspects you cannot. For example, please raise your right hand and hold it in the air. Excellent. Now tell me, how did you do that? When you really think about it, an amazingly complex series of events took place over a matter of seconds. To begin with, you used your eyes to read the words on the page, and your brain decoded them and interpreted them as a request. You thought momentarily and then decided that you would play along and raise your arm as requested. Somehow, in an incredibly complex series of electrical and chemical events and muscle contractions, you raised your arm in a coordinated fashion.

Now, let's try another one. Do me a favor, warm up your hands approximately ten degrees, slow your heart rate down five beats per minute, and decrease the muscle tension in your forehead by five millivolts. Crazy, you say. I say not. After a few short biofeedback sessions, you will be able to do these as easily as raising your arm. How could this be possible, you ask? Because contrary to what you may believe, all your bodily processes can be brought under voluntary control, including heart rate, blood pressure, muscle tension, skin electrical activity, and even brain activity. Biofeedback training essentially makes you the boss and puts you in charge of your physiology. You become the person making choices about how you wish to react.

Biofeedback is a simple technique that any motivated person can master. Typically, you work with a feedback therapist who custom designs a biofeedback relaxation program for you, targeting your specific areas of distress. Training is usually done while you lie comfortably in a recliner. Relaxing images such as warm beaches, open fields, mountains, or images of a special room in your house are used to train your physiology. Auditory and sometimes visual feedback is given as your muscles relax and blood flow improves. Gradually, you learn to voluntarily initiate these positive physiological changes.

I suggest you seek out a therapist certified by the Biofeedback Certification Institute of America. These are individuals who have received specialized training and supervision and have demonstrated competence in this technique.

Hypnosis

Hypnosis is a technique that places you in a state that can best be described as one of heightened suggestibility. This means that when hypnotized, you will accept suggestions about feelings and behavior and incorporate them into your mind. For example, once you are hypnotized, the hypnotist may tell you that each time you see an acne lesion, the act of applying an acne medication will elicit a warm sensation in the skin and an internal feeling of relief. This idea can then be incorporated as a *posthypnotic suggestion*, meaning that subsequently, without any active effort or attention on your part, you actually experience the pleasant sensations and feelings of relief as you apply your acne medications. The association of these positive reactions with your application of skincare medications will make caring for the skin more pleasant and increase the likelihood that you will regularly use your medications.

Guided imagery is often incorporated by hypnotists. While you are in this state of heightened suggestibility, vividly described images can alter your physiological activity. For example, decreased skin itching and burning, decreased heart rate, lowered blood pressure, decreased pain, decreased anxiety, decreased muscle tension, and increased optimism can all be easily achieved. These benefits can often be sustained with posthypnotic suggestions. The improvements in physiology can be helpful in decreasing overall skin irritability and inflammation.

There are many methods that are used to induce a hypnotic state. Guided imagery techniques are sometimes used, such as the classic "You are getting very sleepy . . ." There are innumerable variations that make reference to states of comfort and receptivity, such as "You are drifting slowly into a relaxed state" or "You are sinking comfortably into a deep and restful state." Sometimes, repetitive phrases are employed, or you may be asked to concentrate on a specific object, place, or word. The final common path is a focused state of calm and relaxation in which suggestions can be readily accepted.

Contrary to popular misconception, you will not do anything while under hypnosis that violates your moral and ethical beliefs or desires. However, a hypnotist can get you to perform certain seemingly out-of-character behaviors by altering your perceptions of reality while you are in a hypnotic trance. For example, the hypnotist could tell you that rather than being in a public place, you are actually alone at home in your bedroom, having just returned from a wonderful evening out with friends. The hypnotist may then make a suggestion that you take off your clothes and lie on the table (which has been designated as your bed) and curl up and go to sleep. You may then willingly remove your clothes and, without any inhibition, lie down on the table—believing it is your bed—and go to sleep. Stage hypnotists, to the delight of the audience, commonly use this type of manipulation of perception.

Clearly, much can be accomplished with this amazing tool working in concert with the power of the mind. A professional, therapeutic hypnotist will have your best interest in mind and will not manipulate you in a negative way. Only appropriately trained and certified practitioners should perform this treatment. Many licensed health-care providers perform hypnosis, including physicians, psychologists, social workers, and others with appropriate training. It's a good idea to get a referral from a qualified professional and to check the hypnotist's credentials.

POSITIVE SELF-TALK: COGNITIVE RESTRUCTURING

In this section, we'll return to an idea I introduced in chapter 6: Your thoughts determine your feelings. All too often, you may find yourself feeling angry, anxious, and sad. Sometimes, for no apparent reason, you simply feel out of sorts. You know what I am referring to—that really crummy feeling like you want to crawl out of your skin. These unpleasant feelings are often accompanied by a collection of negative thoughts. These negative thoughts are actually an ongoing dialogue that you produce within your own head. This internal self-talk can cause or fuel a wide array of negative emotions.

For example, a common internal dialogue in response to an acne breakout is as follows. *I can't believe I am breaking out now. This will ruin everything. Everyone will be staring at me and thinking I am some kind of hideous freak. I have the worst luck. Everything always goes wrong for me. I really am a loser.* Of course, by the end of that self-deprecating tirade, anyone would feel depressed and miserable.

However, it doesn't have to play out that way. A different internal dialogue is possible. Let's compare your acne to the following scenarios. Suppose you were just told you had a terminal illness and had only three months to live. Or what if you were involved in a very serious car accident and had both legs severed above your knees? Now, compare that to your acne breakout that has occurred right before a business meeting or party. Given this comparison, you may conclude that you are pretty lucky to only have acne. You may at that point have an internal dialogue that is actually telling you how lucky you are to have a non-life-threatening condition that can be controlled or cured. Now, rather than feeling depressed and miserable, you are feeling happy and relieved.

My point is that your emotional responses to the events and people in your life can be changed and you can bring them under your voluntary control. They can be modified and modulated so that you need not feel so upset, angry, or ugly in response to skin problems or other life events. Replacing some of your negative, sometimes irrational, and self-deprecating internal dialogue with more positive and rational self-talk can decrease the frequency and intensity of your negative emotional responses. In so doing, you will be happier and less stressed, and your body will therefore be less likely to release stress hormones and inflammatory neuropeptides. These changes may result in less acne and less inflammation in the skin.

The Trap of Assumption

If you are like most people, you probably feel very self-conscious when your acne is more active. To make matters worse, people often feel free to make comments about acne and other skin imperfections. Now comes the really ugly part. Since you feel self-conscious and unattractive because of your acne, you begin to embrace a set of assumptions about the thoughts and behavior of others. If they are looking closely at you as you speak, you assume that they are focusing on those miserable and unsightly acne lesions. On the other hand, if they are not looking at you, you assume that they are so repulsed that they cannot bear to look.

This circular trap of assumptions guarantees that you lose. Largely independent of how others respond, you have created a set of assumptions that reinforce your belief that acne is a horrible, life-limiting burden. This perpetuates a cycle of negative self-appraisals that lead to increasingly negative emotional and physical reactions such as sadness, anxiety, anger, lethargy, fatigue, and hopelessness.

Recall from chapter 6 the premise of cognitive behavioral therapy: It is not the events in your life that determine your feelings; it is your thoughts about those events. Emotional happiness and healthy physiology require that you examine and challenge your assumptions. Two specific aspects of your thinking need to be considered. First, you need to examine your assumptions about what people actually notice about your skin and, moreover, what it is that you assume they think when they see your flawed skin. Second, you need to identify what you say to yourself in response to your assumptions about others, because it is this self-talk that can lead you to experience negative and stressful feelings.

EXERCISE 8.4:
EXAMINING YOUR ASSUMPTIONS

Please complete the following sentences. Be as honest as you possibly can.

I assume that when people look at my face, they are thinking that

Because I believe that other people think these things about me, I think

Because I believe that other people think these things about me, I feel

Now you have a great opportunity to examine, evaluate, and change your thoughts and emotional reactions. It does not matter whether or not your assumptions are correct. The truth is, more often than not, other people are not particularly interested in, or aware of, your imperfections. Usually, they are self-absorbed with their own concerns. Even if they are, you don't have to allow others to control your inner emotional experiences.

Examining your thoughts and feelings that you wrote in response to this exercise illustrates the power of your assumptions. If your self-talk is that you are ugly, repulsive, and unacceptable because of your acne and this is an awful thing, then of course you will feel terrible. On the other hand, challenging your assumptions affords you the opportunity to change your self-talk. Instead of allowing your assumptions to elicit negative and anxiety-provoking self-talk, why not go back and modify your answers to reflect more positive assumptions? For example:

I assume that when people look at my face, they are

■ *not really looking at me at all because they are preoccupied with their own stuff.*

■ *noticing my eyes, lips, and words and responding to the messages they are sending.*

■ *staring at my acne or acne scars and thinking something ranging from* Gee, she has some acne *to* Oh wow, what a mess her face is!

The reality is, you can assume all you like, but you will never know for sure what anyone else is actually thinking. Even if they tell you, they may be lying. Therefore, trying to prove or disprove the validity of your assumptions is a useless quest. The solution is to accept the fact that others will think what they will. You do not have the power to change that. You do have the power to avoid the trap of assumption by carefully choosing and practicing more positive and healthful self-talk. You must tell yourself that your self-worth and happiness are not dependent upon the approval of others. The presence or absence of acne or acne scarring need not determine your happiness.

The Trap of "Shoulds" and "Musts"

Filling your internal dialogues with unrealistic expectations of others and yourself lays the foundation for emotional unhappiness. We all compile long lists of "shoulds" and "musts" that reflect our irrational internal dialogue. These are akin to assumptions about what other people are thinking, and they're just as damaging.

■ Sean

Sean, a very frustrated acne sufferer, frequently told me that he should have perfect skin because no one else in his family had acne. He announced to me during an office visit that he must have clear skin within three weeks and he could not stand putting up with his acne for one week longer. He concluded that living with acne was an awful thing and that it would be a major catastrophe in his life if the acne persisted. "Awfulizing" and "catastrophizing" are a natural consequence of these types of internal dialogues. *If I am not acne free by the end of the month, that would be awful, a catastrophe, and I can't stand even the thought of it* is an illustration of these types of self-defeating thoughts. Once events are put into the categories of awful and catastrophic, the resulting emotional reactions must be strong and very negative.

Sean worked with a cognitive behavioral therapist and replaced his negative self-talk with a healthier and more rational internal dialogue. The therapist asked Sean to write down all the thoughts he had surrounding his acne. He was asked to finish incomplete sentences such as *My acne makes me feel . . . , Because I have acne my life is . . . , I can't stand my acne because . . . , People think that I have acne because . . . ,* and *Acne is the worst thing that ever happened to me because . . .* He became aware that it was not his acne that made him feel so badly; rather, it was his awfulizing and catastrophizing self-talk about how horrible it was that he had acne.

Let me be clear about cognitive behavioral interventions. They are not about living a life of Pollyanna stories, pretending that all is rosy and wonderful. That would certainly diminish the seriousness of acne and the negative reality of living with it. The cognitive behavioral school of psychology recognizes and validates the seriousness and realities of the events in your life and your concerns about them. Embracing the challenge of modifying your internal dialogues does not imply that you reduce your efforts or modify your goal of attaining clear skin.

The goal of cognitive restructuring is to identify and challenge your self-talk. Replacing these negative and extreme thoughts with more positive and realistic ones can lead to very substantial and positive changes in your emotions. These changes will definitely improve the quality of your life and probably lead to better skin.

An important point here is that you are probably often unaware of your self-talk. Your self-talk can be identified by examining exactly what you are thinking when you feel a strong negative emotional reaction. Ask yourself, is it an absolute truth that you can never be happy or comfortable with your complexion until the acne scars on your face are completely gone? That deeply held belief or conclusion must by definition be based on your internal dialogue telling you that scars are awful and terrible, capable of ruining your life. In comparison, imagine that you had only one eye, no lips, and jagged, sunken scars covering 95 percent of your face. Now, how unacceptable are the actual imperfections that you see in the mirror? This may sound simplistic, but there is a reality basis to these comparisons.

I agree that your problems are unpleasant, frustrating, and perhaps truly unfair. But they are not so awful that you need punish your body and soul by reacting with extreme and miserable emotions. Choose instead to work toward happiness. Work on changing your self-talk that is causing strong and negative emotional reactions. Work on the task of identifying those things on your skin and in your life that are changeable. Set concrete and attainable goals. Then begin by taking action to move toward these goals when possible. If you, like most people, cannot change all the things that bother you, then reexamine your remaining negative self-talk and free yourself of the emotional burdens. Let your brain wag your emotional tail in a positive way. You need not be a helpless victim of negative self-talk.

CONSIDERING MEDICATION

While I am fundamentally opposed to the unnecessary use of oral medications, there are definitely times when the selective use of antianxiety and antidepressant medications can be tremendously helpful. These medications can help diminish sad and negative feelings, decrease persistent and intrusive obsessive thoughts, and increase energy levels. They tend to blunt the intensity of anxiety and other uncomfortable stress responses, making day-to-day activities less stressful. Antidepressant and antianxiety medications may also decrease the release of stress hormones and inflammatory neuropeptides, thereby making the skin less reactive.

How Antianxiety and Antidepressant Medications Work

Medications that can improve mood or decrease anxiety are generally classified as either antidepressants or antianxiety agents. These medications exert their many positive effects by restoring certain brain chemicals, or *neurotransmitters,* to normal levels. Neurotransmitters are chemical messengers in the brain that are released at the junction between communicating nerve endings, or *synapses.* Thoughts, mood, and actions are all—at least to some degree—mediated by these brain chemicals. Neurotransmitters can become depleted due to genetic predisposition, life stresses, or both. When neurotransmitter levels are low, a wide range of symptoms can occur, such as anxiety, depression, lethargy, difficulties in completing tasks, irritability, obsessional thoughts, compulsive activities, pain, and sleep and appetite disturbance, just to name a few. Antianxiety and antidepressant medications increase neurotransmitter levels either by fostering the release of more neurotransmitters or by preventing them from being reabsorbed. There are three main neurotransmitters that are affected by these medications: *serotonin, norepinephrine,* and *dopamine.* Each of these neurotransmitters, either alone or in combination, can have powerful effects on your moods.

When serious depression or debilitating anxiety is present, the decision regarding whether to take an antidepressant or antianxiety medication is very straightforward. The symptoms are obvious and their impact on your happiness and functioning cannot be denied. It's possible, though, that you could substantially benefit from one of these medications even though you have only modest neurotransmitter depletion and don't think of yourself as being depressed or unusually anxious. The symptoms of modest neurotransmitter depletion are often subtle. Reduced enthusiasm, decreased energy, decreased libido, irritability, and distraction are common manifestations and unfortunately often dismissed as "normal aging." Depletion of neurotransmitters can be a gradual process. Therefore, the changes in mood and perception that occur are gradual as well as subtle. These insidious changes eventually manifest as a generalized "blah" feeling in which life seems to have lost some of its luster or shine.

The response to antidepressant and antianxiety medications can be surprising. People often describe a return of positive feelings and state that they feel more like themselves again. Use of these medications can also substantially augment the benefits you gain from stress management techniques. Progressive muscle relaxation, guided imagery, biofeedback training, hypnosis, yoga, and tai chi all can be practiced more easily when neurotransmitter levels are normal.

Common Antidepressant Medications

Antidepressant medications can be helpful for depression, anxiety, and intrusive-obsessive thoughts. Commonly prescribed antidepressant medications such as Prozac (fluoxetine), Zoloft (sertraline), Paxil (paroxetine), Lexapro (escitalopram), and Celexa (citalopram) are *selective serotonin reuptake inhibitors* and mostly affect levels of serotonin. Remeron (mirtazapine), Wellbutrin (bupropion), and Effexor (venlafaxine) have greater effects on norepinephrine and dopamine. Your physician will choose an agent based upon your most troublesome symptoms and your other psychological and medical needs. There is no single agent that has been shown to be definitely superior; the one that works well for you may not be effective for another person. Thus, if you do not achieve the benefits that you had hoped for with one agent, trying another will probably work well.

Common Antianxiety Medications

Antianxiety medications include the benzodiazepine and nonbenzodiazepine agents. *Benzodiazepines* belong to the group of medicines called *central nervous system depressants,* medicines that slow down the nervous system. These agents are quick acting, often sedating, and can be helpful for short-term management of anxiety. Benzodiazepines can be addicting, causing problems with both dependence and withdrawal. Therefore, they should not be used as a long-term treatment to relieve nervousness or tension caused by the stress of everyday life. Klonopin (clonazepam) and Xanax (alprazolam) are examples of commonly prescribed benzodiazepines. These are agents with a relatively short half-life, meaning that they are metabolized and cleared relatively quickly from the body. Morning sedation can be minimized if an agent with a shorter half-life is taken at bedtime.

Nonbenzodiazepines such as BuSpar (buspirone) are preferable since they are nonaddicting. They can be used for long-term management of anxiety. Their onset of action is not rapid like that of benzodiazepines; two to three weeks are usually necessary before benefits are appreciated.

■ Kathy

Many people who suffer from depression do not necessarily feel sad and consequently don't think of themselves as depressed. Kathy's story illustrates this point. Kathy is a forty-five-year-old who came to see me because of her menopausal acne. She had not had a menstrual period in over a year and noticed that with each passing month, her acne seemed to be getting worse. Her acne, together with hair loss on the scalp and new dark hair on her face, was making her increasingly reclusive. She found herself constantly searching for excuses to avoid social situations, and she began to feel chronically fatigued. Kathy's husband was very upset by her change in attitude and behavior and sarcastically suggested she change her name to I Don't Feel Like It.

When I asked Kathy whether she thought it was possible that she might be depressed, she shook her head and said, "No, I'm just getting old."

All too often, depression is misinterpreted as a normal part of aging. After much explanation and cajoling, I convinced Kathy to try a low dose of Zoloft. Within three weeks, Kathy began to feel more like her "old self." Her energy level increased, and her interest in going out and being with other people returned. Her acne and hair loss improved, and her intimacy with her husband was restored.

While many of these possible benefits do sound appealing, side effects are sometimes encountered. Some find these medications to be stimulating, while others find them to be sedating. Sometimes, sexual side effects such as decreased desire and difficulty in achieving orgasm can be seen. These are usually easily improved by a change in dose or change in medication. Some people are quick to abandon a medication at the first occurrence of bothersome side effects. This can be a mistake, because they stop before the many emotional benefits can be realized.

EXERCISE 8.5: CONSIDERING MEDICATION

Determining whether an antidepressant or antianxiety medication is appropriate for you is not necessarily an easy or black-and-white decision. Affirmative answers to some of the following questions indicate that it may be beneficial for you to initiate a discussion about antidepressant or antianxiety medication with your primary care practitioner or dermatologist.

☐ true ☐ false   Sadness and depressing thoughts fill a large part of my day or night.

☐ true ☐ false   I don't seem to have as much energy as I used to.

☐ true ☐ false   Pleasant things like food, flowers, and intimacy no longer interest me as they used to.

☐ true ☐ false   I am having trouble with sleeping either too much or too little.

☐ true   ☐ false   I can't seem to escape intrusive and troubling thoughts.

☐ true   ☐ false   I often feel extremely nervous and jittery.

☐ true   ☐ false   I suffer from panic attacks (sudden and intense feelings of dread or impending doom, racing thoughts, rapid heart rate, tremulousness).

☐ true   ☐ false   I often pick at my skin.

☐ true   ☐ false   I am excessively preoccupied with my skin.

☐ true   ☐ false   I feel very fearful in social situations.

In this chapter, I've introduced several methods to modify your stress responses. I encourage you to learn and practice these techniques to help you better cope with stress, anxiety, and depression. This can help improve your acne as well as your quality of life.

9

Enhancing Your Social Life

Let's begin with what I call the "when I'm fixed" paradox. Perhaps you have a secret internal set of rules that determine what changes must be in place before you are allowed to be happy and actively engaged in your life. Another name for these rules is the "I'll be happy when" straitjacket. I call this a "straitjacket" because essentially this way of thinking leaves you tied up and removed from the world of living until your criteria are met. Therefore, if "fixed" means totally free of acne, you must put your life on hold until you have reached that goal. Meanwhile, the stress, anger, misery, and loneliness of being a spectator of life as it passes you by often leads to worsening of your skin problem. And so the vicious cycle continues. Bad skin, bad emotions, bad physiological reactions, more bad skin.

It is incumbent upon you to make a bold decision, and that decision is the choice of living. That means deciding and choosing to live life now, as you wish it to be, whether your skin is free of acne lesions and scars or rife with imperfection. While I do not deny that there are genuine social difficulties and possible rejections and missed opportunities that can result from visible acne lesions, choosing to avoid life because of your acne guarantees lost opportunities. The more times you push yourself to actively engage in life, the less impact acne is likely to have on your psyche and happiness. It does not matter whether it is attending a book club, religious service, night class, or after-work happy hour or volunteering to read books to children or work in a soup kitchen. It is simply about being connected to life and the living and doing something with meaning. "Meaning" implies something that interests you, stimulates you, helps others, or helps you. There need not be a concrete goal or measurable ending. It is about reaching, experiencing, and touching your world.

ACNE AND SEXUALITY

Many of my acne patients tell me that acne significantly inhibits their willingness to seek out intimacy and their ability to comfortably enjoy it. Self-consciousness about your acne or acne scars and any associated physical discomfort can make the prospect of being touched very upsetting and anxiety provoking. You may actually be menaced by images that you have conjured up in your mind. For example, Gina, a longtime acne sufferer, told me that she would recoil whenever anyone tried to touch her face because of a troubling image that always flashed in her mind. She pictured an exaggerated look of repulsion and disgust on the face of a stranger as he touched her face. This was a look that signified extreme rejection, a confirmation of her feelings of ugliness and disfigurement.

What a terrible irony. From birth to death, we all need to be touched. Gentle touch communicates tenderness, caring, and love. Gina's belief that she was unattractive compelled her to withdraw and even run from the very touch that she so badly needed and even craved. Can you relate to Gina? If so, let me show you how things can get even worse and you can unintentionally create a self-fulfilling prophecy.

Imagine this scenario. You find yourself increasingly attracted to a wonderful new person who happens to have acne. After what seems like an eternity, that special moment finally comes when words are interrupted by a moment of silence and sustained eye contact. Those wonderful and hard-to-explain feelings begin to emerge.

You can suddenly feel your heart beating, your chest tightens, and butterflies fill your stomach. After taking a deep breath, you gather your courage and apprehensively seize the moment. You reach gently to touch the person's face, but your anticipation is abruptly shattered when the person withdraws and turns away. Hurt and filled with feelings of rejection, you immediately withdraw. Your warmth and tenderness are quickly replaced with what appears only as cool detachment. The acne sufferer, head still turned, is acutely aware of your change in demeanor, certain that the change occurred because you came close enough to be repulsed by the acne.

The self-fulfilling prophecy is complete. Self-loathing makes the acne sufferer unable to accept intimacy. Inability to accept intimacy is interpreted by the suitor as rejection. Rejection leads to hurt, which leads to physical and emotional withdrawal on the part of the suitor. The self-loathing of the acne sufferer intensifies.

Now imagine the implications of this scenario in the intimacy of the bedroom. Everyone is self-conscious about his or her body and sexual prowess. Thus, when the acne sufferer withdraws from a sexual encounter due to self-consciousness, the partner inevitably interprets the withdrawal as lack of interest and desire. Dejected and certain that the problem lies with his own lack of desirability and adequacy, the suitor responds in an angry and aloof manner to protect the bruised, fragile ego. Both partners engage in damage control, withdrawing further, only confirming and worsening the miserable feelings. Meaningful intimacy and desire for sex are sacrificed.

Foreplay starts long before you enter the bedroom. Each partner needs to feel acceptable and accepted. Acne really is not the issue. Inability to accept acne and accept intimacy in spite of acne is the issue. Sex is a funny thing. It's not about whether you have clear skin or a perfect body. It's about accepting yourself and others. With acceptance comes freedom—the freedom to accept and give freely without self-consciousness or appraisal. Then you are free to enjoy intimacy.

CHOOSING PERSONHOOD OVER PERFECTION

I wish perfection on no one, including you. Perfection is a precarious and passing state from which you can only fall. People with perfect skin or perfect bodies are always on the verge of imperfection. It is inevitable: they will break out, age, and gain weight. Their pores will enlarge, hair will gray, breasts will sag, and wrinkles will form.

Guess what else. Since they often have learned to define their self-worth based on their "perfect" physical beauty, the imperfections can be devastating for them, creating emotional havoc.

I've got a better choice. How about learning to live happily surrounded by your perfectly unique, imperfect wrapping? Imperfection allows for individuality and personhood. Personhood is your cognitive and emotional neighborhood in the world. It is composed of the people and things that are important to you as an individual. Personhood is largely independent of your physical attributes. It is about you, the person—a unique person with interests, abilities, aspirations, fears, and kooky thoughts that are yours alone. The inner you, that part of you that has your own unique thoughts and feelings, is not a person who cares to conform to some societally dictated, cookie-cutter image of cloned Barbie dolls. The inner you is a person who can choose to live as a happy, imperfect person. This does not imply that you ignore styles and trends that are personally appealing to you or necessary for work and social obligations. The irony of chasing perfection is that it often requires that people relinquish qualities that distinguish them as individuals, the very qualities that make others choose them as their employees, friends, and life partners.

RUN, WHILE THERE'S STILL TIME

Run where, you ask. Really, the question is whether you should run toward or away from life. "Run, while there's still time" conjures up images of someone desperately trying to escape from harm before time runs out. Implied in this phrase is the concept that action is necessary to avoid harm. You must take action before time runs out. Passivity or inaction only guarantees that you will lose and the clock will keep ticking.

There is still time. Whether you are eighteen or seventy-eight, you can make the choice to run toward life and the living. Don't allow yourself to be discouraged or dissuaded by negative thoughts. Now is the time for action. Seek out legitimate care for your acne or acne scars while simultaneously running toward the people and activities that will give your life purpose and meaning. This may mean pursuing a job, career, education, or new friend. It may mean volunteering in a hospital, library, or house of worship. It may mean reading a book, planting a garden, or getting a pet.

Many of my patients find it useful to write a to-do list. You know, one of those lists of groceries to buy or all-important household chores to be done. Well, this one is a bit different. It is the "stuff I really want to do before it's too late" list. This list can really help you focus on the things that bring you pleasure and give your life meaning and purpose.

EXERCISE 9.1: THE "STUFF I REALLY WANT TO DO BEFORE IT'S TOO LATE" LIST

- get better control of my acne

- improve my acne scars

- _____

- _____

- _____

- _____

- _____

- _____

THE PIE OF LIFE

Apple pie, cherry pie, lemon meringue pie, whichever is your pleasure. How about a slice? Would you like a big slice or a merely a sliver?

The pie of life represents all the possible social interactions that you can have in your life. It is the people, places, and things that fill your world and surround you. Family relationships, platonic friendships, romantic friendships, work or business relationships, and sports relationships, to name only a few, are all part of your social world.

Other relationships in your house of worship, community service organization, art group, bridge class, adult education class, and so on are all slices of this pie of life. Inevitably, the filling and size of the slices change as your life evolves.

EXERCISE 9.2: YOUR PIE OF LIFE

Take a look at the sample pie and the percent of life each slice represents. On a piece of paper, draw a big circle. Now ask yourself, how would you label your pie of life? Is there the right number of slices? Is your life varied enough, or is it lacking in variation? Are you happy with the percent of your life occupied by each slice?

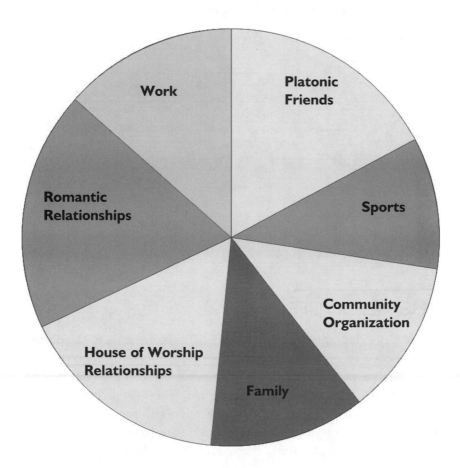

If there are obvious changes that you would like to make, get out the pie cutter and begin the task of serving up slices that are right for you at this time in your life. Your pie of life is an ever evolving creation. You can change the filling and serving sizes as your tastes change. Sometimes the crust gets stale and the filling distasteful; that is the cue to bake a new pie. Look to new people and places for the ingredients.

10

Living Well with Acne: Having a Full and Meaningful Life

Whether you currently have acne, have phantom acne, or are living with the physical and emotional scars from acne, the solution to the problem of acne involves a dual approach. While learning to better manage your acne, your other job is to learn how to live your life well and in a meaningful way.

THE POWER OF SMALL, INCREMENTAL CHANGES

We are a society obsessed with big. We want big houses, big diamonds, big cars, and huge successes. We seek out the big sale, attend the huge event, and look for colossal savings. Given this perspective, we often are unable to appreciate the enormous value of small changes in our lives. Small, incremental changes can bring tremendous emotional benefit. For example, I and my colleagues performed a study (Fried and Cash 1998) in our center that demonstrated that simply using a therapeutic-strength alpha hydroxy acid on the face for twelve weeks resulted in dramatic emotional benefit. As expected, patients had modest improvement in fine wrinkles, skin texture, and uneven pigmentation. What we did not expect were the statistically significant emotional benefits that patients achieved. Participants in the study felt better about themselves, were more satisfied with their bodies, and felt more satisfied sexually. How could the simple application of a topical lotion make such a difference?

The answer lies in the power of incremental change. You don't need to see dramatic change in order to be happy. In fact, too much change too quickly can have the opposite effect. Large, rapid changes can be frightening and disruptive to your psychological equilibrium. Small changes elicit optimism. Optimism allows you to answer those negative subconscious thoughts about aging, unattractiveness, decline, and deterioration. The modest benefits of the alpha hydroxy acid lotion allowed study participants to respond to thoughts such as *I'm not what I used to be, I can't stand those scars and spots,* and *It's all downhill from here* with more positive answers such as *I actually look better than I did three months ago* and *Things are getting better.*

The take-home message is that as soon as you initiate any proactive step to improve your skin and life, the positive emotions will follow. Simply stated, just do something, begin the forward process of change, and then you can begin to shine your own spotlight of positivity on your life and your accomplishments. This is more than a game of semantics. Choosing to focus on positive changes, no matter how small, can have huge emotional benefits.

A PROGRAM FOR A HAPPY AND MEANINGFUL LIFE

A simple daily program can change your life. It can give you more emotional freedom and happiness and diminish your tendencies toward self-deprecation, anxiety, and unnecessary sadness. Positive thoughts and feelings coupled with increased energy can enhance your ability to enjoy life, feel more positive emotions, think more clearly, focus better, laugh more, and live better. Before I explain the program, I want to introduce you to Cindy, an individual who desperately needed to join the program and embark on the road to inner beauty and freedom.

■ Cindy

Cindy, an overweight and somewhat disheveled thirty-six-year-old woman, came to our center with what physicians call a "chief complaint" of worsening acne. Doctors always specify a chief complaint because it allows us to focus on the main symptom causing a patient distress. We are taught in medical school that the chief complaint can sometimes be the outer sign of a more serious underlying problem. This was exactly the situation for Cindy.

Despite her unkempt, overweight, and sad appearance, it was obvious to me that Cindy was attractive. She told me that until two years earlier, she had been a relatively trim, meticulously groomed, happy person who—with the exception of a few premenstrual breakouts—always had great skin. She had liked her job, was happily married, and enjoyed the challenges of raising her two young children.

But Cindy told me that somehow, gradually, she felt as though "things began to slip away." Her husband traveled often, and Cindy frequently functioned as a single parent. She had almost no free time, no time for exercise, and her meals often were frozen dinners or prepared entrées from the supermarket. Her house seemed to her to be in a constant state of disarray and confusion. Cindy's growing feelings of fatigue and frustration sometimes were overwhelming. Most people she knew seemed to have it much more together than she did. They seemed happier, did more things, and had many more material possessions than she did. She increasingly envied their lives and felt disappointed and cheated by her own.

Then, out of nowhere, her skin began to break out with deep, inflamed cystic lesions. Cindy's acne only worsened her already miserable feelings. It felt to her like the last straw. The months seemed to pass by quickly, leaving only a blur of unfinished chores and self-loathing thoughts. What happened to the happy, together person she used to be? Why did everything feel so meaningless? Cindy concluded that this was middle age, the price of getting older.

Wrong, wrong, wrong! Life need not lose its shine, and excitement need not lessen as time goes on. The opportunities to live life fully, enjoy each day, and savor the moment never must diminish. Cindy became trapped, helplessly sinking into the quicksand of life. She lost her perspective about what was really important. Her relationship with her husband and children had become overshadowed by all the overwhelming details of her life. Her self-worth had been eroded. There was no energy and motivation left for living and loving.

Cindy needed more than improvement in her acne. Eliminating her acne alone would not have freed her from her internal turmoil and liberated her to become a happy person. Cindy needed to accept herself as a normal person with flaws and limitations, and define what was necessary and important for her to achieve a truly meaningful existence. She needed to relinquish the patterns of thought and behavior that had prevented her from finding her inner beauty.

There are two important messages in Cindy's story. The first is that negative emotional and behavioral changes can be very insidious. Changes can creep up on you, unnoticed, unsolicited, and unwelcome. Cindy certainly did not create a plan in which her happiness and her inclination to take care of herself would be yanked away from her. The demands of life, her fatigue, her husband's absences, and the changes in her skin and body all played a part. She was unaware of how unhappy and how neglectful of herself she had become. The second important message is that everything cannot be fixed all at once and that all cannot be made perfect by any single change. Simply prescribing medical treatments for Cindy's acne would not resolve her fundamental unhappiness. What Cindy needed was a comprehensive change program that addressed not just her skin problems but her entire approach to life and her sense of herself.

THE STEP PROGRAM

STEP is an acronym for a four-part program for positive life change. The S is for the major stressors in your life. The T is for targeting specific stressors for change. The E is for envisioning your life as it might be if that stress were modified. The P is for making an identifiable, proactive change in your life.

EXERCISE 10.1: THE STEP PROGRAM

1. Identify Your Stressors

Begin by making a list of the things that cause you significant stress in your life. Included on the list may be your acne, acne scars, other aspects of your body you're dissatisfied with (nose, lips, wrinkles, breasts), dietary habits, exercise routine (or lack thereof), weight, significant other, family member, job, children, or overall health. For now, don't worry about the order of the items in your list. Just jot them down as you think of them.

-
-
-
-
-
-
-
-
-
-

Now prioritize your stressors, identifying those that stress you the most and those that stress you the least. Rewrite the list above in the space below, arranging the items in order from most stressful (1) to least stressful (10).

1.

2.

3.

4.

5.

6.

7.

8.

9.

10.

The next step is to separate your stressors into two categories, those that there is some hope of changing and those that there is little or no hope of changing.

Stressors I can change   **Stressors I cannot change**

The stressors for which you believe there is some hope for change are the ones you will target and attempt to change. Those that you are certain are not amenable to change are the ones you will work to accept, at least for now. If peaceful acceptance is not possible, the goal will be to respond with as little negative emotional and physical energy as possible.

2. Target a Stressor to Change

The next step is to move on to the T of the STEP program. The T asks you to target a stressor from your "Stressors I can change" list.

For example, you may choose to target your acne. The ultimate goal is to be free of acne, and the short-term goal is to experience acne as less stressful.

3.   Envision Your Life with That Stressor Modified

Next is the E in the STEP program. Envision how much better you would feel if your acne were better and you felt more in control of its occurrence and your emotional reactions to it. Using this model, any proactive step you take to better manage your acne should reduce stress and enhance your sense of optimism and control.

4.   Proactively Change That Stressor

Now, here comes the P for the proactive part. Specifically, each time you gently cleanse your skin and apply a topical acne medication or herbal preparation, you can and should allow yourself to experience a reduction in stress. Talk to your acne lesions and negotiate a peace accord. The rules of the accord are as follows: *I wish you gone, but I refuse to allow your presence the power to ruin my happiness.*

You can apply the same four-step program to other stressors on your list of things that could be changed. For example, suppose you identify your commute, which involves an hour-long drive in very heavy traffic, as a major source of stress and decide that you want to try to change it somehow. You envision yourself arriving home at the end of the day feeling relaxed, energetic, and ready to enjoy the evening with your family. You decide to try borrowing audiobooks from the library and listening to them on your car stereo, rather than listening to the traffic reports on the radio over and over or using your cell phone to check your office voicemail. You discover that in fact this works well for you, especially because you don't otherwise have time to read as much as you'd like to. You become absorbed in the story you're listening to, and traffic delays simply mean that you get to hear more of it. When you arrive in your driveway and turn off the car, you feel as though you're putting down a favorite book. You are surprised to discover that your commute has actually become a source of pleasure.

Setting Attainable Goals

How will you know when you've successfully accomplished the changes you set out to make? Concrete, observable, and realistically attainable short-term goals are the basis of the STEP program. Identifiable markers of change are like road signs, reassuring you that you are on the right path to positive change. Without these markers, the task of attaining happiness, improved appearance, and acceptance of self seems too overwhelming and confusing.

Being the Power Broker

The STEP program is very much a program of empowerment. Identifying stressors, targeting ones to change, envisioning your life with those stressors changed or at least causing less stress, and most importantly being proactive is a process of empowerment. You become a power broker, deciding how much of your emotional energy and self-worth will be given over to anyone or anything. It really is a matter of giving yourself the power of choice. Your happiness and minute-to-minute stress can be modified by your thoughts and your choices.

The beauty of the STEP program is how it directs your attention and energy to make real changes in your life. A very important benefit of the program is its strength-building aspect. Each time you use the STEP program and achieve any degree of success, you will gain more confidence in yourself and become stronger and more capable in your ability to handle stress.

Accepting Yourself

A factory defect is an item that has deficiencies in material, workmanship, or function. As such, this item should be returned to the factory, where it should be replaced or fixed to achieve a production standard of excellence or perfection. Quality control engineers spend their lives testing, evaluating, and critiquing the finished products of a manufacturing or production effort.

Human beings are the end product of a production effort. The question is, when looked at critically by a quality control engineer, how do we fare? Well, which do you want first, the good news or the bad news? I'll give you both at once. Based upon objective quality control data, the bad news is that we are all factory defects. We all have imperfect hair, eyes, ears, noses, lips, chins, breasts, arms, waists, buttocks, knees, and toes. Acne, stretch marks, scars, moles, birth-marks, and a plethora of other imperfections are part of all of us. But the bad news is really the good news. Each person—including you—is wonderful, varied, interesting, unique, and lovable. Perfection does not exist. The closer you come to perfection, the bigger the burden of misery.

Therefore, since I hope we agree that you are perfectly imper-fect, your job is to learn to accept yourself. Let me be clear. Accepting yourself does not imply passive acceptance of your physical, emo-tional, and spiritual state "as is." Accepting yourself implies sincerely and genuinely realizing that you are a physically, emotionally, and spiritually imperfect, flawed being capable of rotten and unacceptable thoughts, feelings, and impulses. Accepting yourself recognizes that you are always seeking to improve yourself. You are a work in prog-ress. The beauty of a work in progress is the acknowledgment that change and evolution are lifelong processes. Therefore, it is essential to recognize that acceptance of self and desire for change are not contradictory principles. Accepting yourself simply requires that you allow yourself periods of happiness and contentment even though you are physically, emotionally, and spiritually imperfect. Without this acceptance, you will most likely be unable to move forward and make meaningful changes in your life.

■ Cindy

Cindy was initially reluctant to accept the concept of the STEP program. She told me that she had no time to address any other issues in her life besides her acne. I agreed with her that her life certainly was busy and the demands of young children, work, and an often-absent husband must be overwhelming. I shared with her my concerns about her per-ception that life had lost its meaning and that things had become a blur. I told her that all human beings feel angry, confused, inadequate, exhausted, overwhelmed, and out of control at various times, but that it is not an inevitable part of the aging process to feel that life has lost its meaning. I specifically inquired about her impulses and thoughts, asking her if she had any thoughts or impulses of hurting herself or anyone else. She vehemently denied any of these fears other than the angry impulses that all parents feel when frustrated by their children and spouse.

After my brief inquiry and short burst of philosophical statements, I told Cindy that we would simply address her acne, as she requested, and consider other aspects of her life at a future time if she so desired. Several seconds later, as I examined the inflammatory lesions on her cheeks, Cindy began to cry. She looked at me, shaking her head slowly from side to side, and said, "It is so much more than my acne."

I smiled and placed my hand gently on her arm. My words to her were simple. "This is a wonderful thing. You don't have to let life go by in a blur, missing all the opportunities for happiness and pleasure that each day offers. You told me that life has become a blur and at times feels meaningless. Today marks the beginning of a new chapter in your life, a chapter with clarity and meaning."

I shared with her that for all of us, each day is often like a roller-coaster ride. There are the highs and the lows, sometimes occurring seconds apart or even simultaneously. I suggested to Cindy that the recipe for happiness involves removing as much emotional baggage as possible. The baggage is composed of thoughts, perceptions, judgments of self and others, and inherited brain chemistry. I explained that thoughts, perceptions, and judgments can be modified by using effective self-help strategies or by working with a competent therapist. Further, I explained how inherited brain chemistry can predispose a person to anxiety, depression, and obsessive tendencies and suggested that, sometimes, taking an antidepressant or antianxiety medication can be absolutely liberating and essential.

Cindy and I decided that the best approach would be for her to begin by adding biofeedback therapy to her standard dermatologic treatment. Cindy worked with the biofeedback therapist at our center. She identified and targeted several other stressors in addition to her acne. Her weight, inactivity, lack of personal time, perfectionist standards, and unrealistic perceptions regarding the competence and happiness of others were targeted as stressors. Following the STEP program, Cindy targeted each of these stressors.

Regarding her weight and inactivity, she envisioned how much better she would feel and ultimately look if she made exercise a part of her daily routine again. Cindy's therapist helped her to envision realistic and easily obtainable goals. Cindy was asked to envision herself walking on the treadmill, beginning with only five minutes each day. She was instructed to focus on her legs, feeling the muscles coming alive and getting stronger. The therapist guided Cindy in placing similar focus on her arms, abdomen, chest, and back. Special attention was paid to her breathing. Cindy was asked to imagine deep, healthful breaths, with each inhalation filling her lungs and body with essential oxygen. Cindy was asked to imagine and experience a sensation of release and tension reduction with each effortless exhalation.

Cindy was able to envision this scenario and imagine these sensations, and she made her proactive move in the STEP program, beginning her treadmill workout the next day. She found the effort minimal but was surprised at how positive and optimistic she felt at the end of her short workout. Envisioning more success and more progress, she imagined and then completed longer and more involved workouts as the weeks progressed. She always kept her focus on the short term, envisioning only activities and feelings that she could readily achieve. As Cindy exercised more and lost more weight, her overall energy level and feelings of well-being increased. The envisioning component of the STEP program was always evolving, allowing for adjustments based upon Cindy's emotional and physical progress.

Cindy also used the STEP program to address her perfectionist standards. She believed that the neatness and orderliness of her house directly reflected her competence as a mother and wife. Despite the fact that Cindy realized the absurdity of this belief system, she found it extremely difficult to deal with the constant mess. Cindy's therapist asked her to envision herself less stressed and less angry despite some mess and disarray in her home. She envisioned herself focusing on the faces of her children or, better still, on some other aspect of her world that was beautiful or in order. She envisioned herself trying to confine more of the mess to certain areas. She decided to create for herself a "neat room" that she could keep locked, allowing her things to remain in order.

Her proactive steps proved helpful. Cindy certainly continued to experience frustration and annoyance, but she noted a substantial decrease in the frequency and intensity of these responses. She began to look at the bigger picture and realized that she could find a small amount of time for herself. She found a neighborhood teenager and hired her one hour per day as a mother's helper. During this hour, Cindy would catch up on chores but also would sometimes take a bath or read a magazine.

Cindy's acne did clear completely. Perhaps as importantly or more importantly, other things about her life became clear as well, allowing her to regain her happiness.

"JUST ONE MORE TIME"

Let me share with you my candy machine philosophy of life. Imagine that you are a candy machine. All day long, people come to you and pull your knobs for their treats. This process can continue indefinitely as long as one crucial event takes place. The candy machine must be restocked regularly, or there will be no more candy to give.

How do you restock your emotional candy machine so that the people in your world can continue to pull your knobs without you running out of treats? The answer lies in achieving a balanced life. Your goal should be to find and embrace a "self-indulgent" activity that brings you pleasure. Daily attempts at stress management are essential.

Most of all, actively search for the child who lives deep down within you. Cultivate "Just one more time!" moments. Anyone who has been around young children knows about these. Whether it's inspired by the amusement park ride, the jump off your knees, or the tickle under the arms, "One more time!" flows from their little mouths even before the heartfelt laughter stops. Children know the secret: fully embrace the joy of the moment, hold it tight, then try your very best to make it last and last. What is the wisdom that these innocent young souls possess? Simply stated, joy is to be sought, savored, and cherished.

Watch children, your own or others. Watch cartoons and silly movies. Try to focus on simple pleasures, and remind yourself to stop and savor the moment. Work on being a child, and you just may find yourself saying, "One more time!"

SHIFTING YOUR PERSPECTIVE

Go with me on this one for a minute. Let's look at acne from a cultural perspective. Suppose you were raised in a different culture, where pimples were a sign of intelligence, strength, wealth, superior genes, and sexual prowess. Now look in the mirror. What assumptions would others make about you if this were the case? In this culture, the lucky ones would welcome the development of acne, since it obviously would bring prestige and attract the envy of others. They would proudly hold their heads high so their pimples could be seen. I reiterate, it is not the occurrence of acne that determines the emotional response but rather the self-talk about the acne.

Am I being absurd in looking at the cultural context to prove that it is not the acne that causes emotions? Suppose that twenty years ago, you had been told that someday, people would proudly show off earrings in their noses, tongues, nipples, and belly buttons. You probably would have told me that I was crazy. Well, maybe so, but have a look around. Indeed, reactions to life events are based in cultural context and in our interpretation of those events.

Unfortunately, our culture does not yet hold acne in high esteem. Acne stinks; about that we agree. But what if you substitute *I hate* and *I can't stand* and *This is awful* with *I am genuinely annoyed and peeved that I have to deal with these pimples. Despite them, I have many things of greater importance in my life, and I refuse to let acne stop me from doing, going, and being a part of life. Moreover, whatever others may think does not have to affect how I feel. Ideally, I would like them to think positively about me, but I refuse to have my emotions raised and lowered like a window shade based on what I think they think or what they say. I am entitled to my own opinions and emotions, and today I choose to think and feel in a healthier and more positive way. I want my body and skin to be happier.*

This does not imply that you are any less motivated to achieve clear skin. Ongoing efforts to attain great skin are separate from taking control of your thoughts and emotions in the here and now. In fact, the better you do with your thoughts and emotions, the better your skin is likely to do.

BECOMING THE APPRAISER

Closely related to the trap of assumptions, which you learned about in chapter 8, is the concept of appraisal. Appraisers are people who get paid to determine the value of a given object. Cars, jewelry, homes, boats, coins, and even animals are given an appraised value or worth. It doesn't stop there. What about people? We too are regularly appraised. Professional athletes, entertainers, business leaders, teachers, salespeople, and politicians are regularly "appraised" for their monetary value and performance.

But who determines the value of your internal happiness, your self-acceptance, your self-worth, and your human worth? These are the things that affect your true happiness and health. Who is the appropriate appraiser of these cherished possessions? The answer to this question is twofold. If you are religious, the ultimate appraiser is God, although your own appraisal of yourself matters, too. If you are not religious, it is you alone. Either way, it is your actions that largely determine your value. You may not be able to change the events in your life, but you can change what you do and how you react.

Don't give away your right to be your own appraiser. Live your life according to the values, interests, passions, and goals you cherish. If you don't know exactly what they are, this is a great opportunity for exploration. The true meaning of happiness in life is living in the moment and experiencing the passion of the search for new meaningful moments. Age, skin blemish, nor infirmity need not stand in the way of the search. See a movie, read a book, visit a bookstore or museum. Take a course, learn to knit, enroll in a yoga class. Call a friend or reach out to make a new one. Get a pet. Say something nice to someone for no reason other than to see the person smile. Hug a loved one. Say "I love you" to someone special. Look closely at someone you haven't really looked at in a long time; rediscovery is fun. Attend a religious service or a community event.

The more you live life, the more positive your appraisals will become. It's a funny thing, but as you become more involved in living life and sharing with others, you will find less time and inclination for making appraisals. Now that is healthy freedom.

IDENTITY THEFT

Much has been written recently about identity theft, a crime in which someone gains access to important personal information about you and uses that information to steal from you. Acne too can be thought of as a robbery of your identity. Allow me to explain.

Your self-image or sense of who you are began its development very early in your life. Observing the delight and fascination apparent on the face of an infant peering endlessly into a mirror shows us the beginning of identity development. At first, it is clear that infants do not realize that the image they see is their own. Gradually, the recognition grows as they make varied expressions and fully enjoy the experience, free of any judgment or negative appraisal. This identity of self is not a fixed or stagnant perception. It continues to evolve throughout the life span. Adolescence is often a nightmarish period with tormenting perceptions of identity. Our human tendency to minimize our positives and embellish and envy those of others fuels the commonly negative self-appraisals.

If your acne started when you were a teenager, it interrupted the development of your identity; if it started when you were an adult, it changed your existing identity. Acne can be perceived as a thief, robbing and assaulting your identity of self. These assaults on your identity may lead you to feel shy, damaged, unlovable, and ugly.

If you have active acne, phantom acne, or acne scars, your identity is that of someone who has acne. Now comes the really important part: How much identity theft will you allow? How much of your personal happiness and positive perceptions of yourself will you allow to be stolen? The answers to these questions are determined by how much you have previously allowed and continue to allow your identity as an acne sufferer to affect you. Are you someone who is displeased and somewhat annoyed by this intrusion? If so, you will continue on with your life largely uninterrupted. In contrast, if you are someone who has allowed the presence of acne to unleash a plethora of negative and catastrophic self-talk, your life will be dramatically affected for the worse. Anger, sadness, anxiety, and withdrawal from life will become your calling card.

Which have you chosen? What do you wish your calling card to read? *It's me, same worthwhile human being, please excuse a few zits*, or would you rather *It's the new me, angry, negative, scarred, miserable, hopeless . . . Stay away.*

It really is your choice. By the way, there is a third choice. Acne does give you the opportunity for a new and improved you. Imperfection, blemish, affliction: all give you the chance to reappraise your life and how you wish to live it from now on.

FIND YOUR EMOTIONAL VIAGRA

The power of positive expectation cannot be overstated. Throughout the history of psychology and medicine, expectation has been shown to powerfully affect emotions, performance, and physiology. An impressive example involves the placebo studies performed on Viagra (sildenafil). Viagra, as you probably know, is a medication used to treat erectile dysfunction in men. As is true for most medications, the effectiveness of the Viagra pill was tested against a placebo pill. A *placebo* is an inactive substance or preparation. The studies on Viagra found that almost 30 percent of the men who took only the placebo pill had the same positive response as those who took the active medication (Physicians' Desk Reference 2005). The effect was not just in their heads. Many of the men who took only the placebo pill had a real and observable series of physiological changes culminating in an erection—simply because they expected the pill to work.

This expectation phenomenon has been seen with many other medications and treatments, proving that for many people, expectancy can substantially affect physiology. I am not just talking about mind over matter; I am emphatically stating that the mind matters.

I encourage you to identify and use your emotional Viagra. It may be an over-the-counter salicylic acid, benzoyl peroxide, or glycolic acid product. It may be green tea, omega-3 oils, flaxseed, chamomile, or a multivitamin. Or, it may be your prescription acne product or antidepressant medication. Regardless of which product you choose, you've gotta believe! The positive emotional and physiological effects can only benefit your body, skin, and happiness.

11

Now It's Your Turn

It is probably obvious to you at this point that healing adult acne is not a simple matter of finding the right miracle acne-fighting product. Because you have read this book, you have become an educated consumer, an advocate for your own health, a person who is better able to make intelligent and logical choices about treating your acne. You can look up the different acne treatments that are available and decide whether they make sense for your acne. You can bring this book or the information provided within to the cosmetic counter, pharmacy, and your skincare provider. Use the book as a reference as you read the labels on over-the-counter products; then make good choices. Use the book to understand the rationale for recommendations made by your dermatologist. You have been well saturated with facts and stories that emphasize the point that true healing often involves finding the correct treatment regimen that complements your unique, individual skin biology and personality. This regimen may include only topical antiacne medications, or it may be a combination of topical and oral medications coupled with vitamins, stress management techniques, assessments of your life and coping strategies, and antidepressant medication.

I encourage you to complete the assessments of your acne and your emotions. I also urge you to consider practicing some of the stress management techniques offered throughout the book. Pay particular attention to the impact acne has had on your skin and your life. The stress management, cognitive restructuring, and life assessment exercises are designed to help you improve both your skin and your life.

HEALING IS A LIFELONG PROCESS

Injuries and subsequent healing are an inevitable part of the life process. Acne lesions, paper cuts, scrapes, splinters, bruises, and lacerations: the skin is subject to an ongoing barrage of insults and attacks. Thankfully, you are a magnificently complex being with an innate capacity to heal. Your job and obligation is to provide a physical and emotional environment that is maximally conducive to health and healing.

Healing is a main thrust of this book. Close inspection of the skin and psyche of every living person will reveal innumerable scars that have accrued as a result of the journey through life. These scars may be viewed by some as flaws and signs of imperfection. I prefer a healthier view, choosing to look at scars as a membership card in the club of life. Scars are evidence of living. Scars themselves rarely interfere with the functioning of a person. However, preoccupation with acne and scars can be crippling. Healing acne lesions and dealing with the scars left by the occurrence of acne is the key to leaving behind burdensome baggage that need not weigh on your happiness.

YOU CAN WIN THE SKIN GAME

You can win the skin game, but winning does not necessarily mean attaining perfect, flawless skin. Perfect skin does not exist in reality. I stare at thousands of faces and bodies each year, many belonging to well-known celebrities. I assure you, perfection is an illusion. It exists only in airbrushed magazine pages and digitally enhanced movie images. Achieving and maintaining perfection is impossible, and the emotional price is unaffordable.

"Perfect people" are miserable, exhausted by their efforts to maintain the illusion of their perfection. They are resentful of others who define them by their perfection and demand that they always live the part. Most movie stars and supermodels eventually burn out, and many turn to alcohol and drugs to alleviate the stress and pain associated with maintaining their supposed perfection. They pay the emotional and physical toll of living in a society that refuses to allow them human flaws. So, as a starting point, be careful of what you envy and wish for.

Real human beings like you and me have imperfect skin with blemishes, blood vessels, dark and light spots, rough texture, visible pores, oil spots, and unwanted hair. Perhaps you can view these imperfections not as an affliction but as a blessing in disguise. As a real living person, you are a wonderfully imperfect being. It is not necessary to live the lie of physical and emotional perfection. You need not live imprisoned by the false illusions portrayed in the media. You can simply strive for good skin, good heart, and good soul. So my definition of winning the skin game is helping you to achieve realistic, healthy skin within which you can live comfortably and interact meaningfully with those in your world.

WHAT WILL BE YOUR EPITAPH?

Epitaphs are those short descriptions of a life often inscribed artfully on a tombstone. *Loving mother, beloved wife, caring father,* or perhaps *cherished friend* are typical inscriptions. Funny, but you never see inscriptions like *great worrier, terrific housekeeper, really organized, had a high-powered job,* or *never had acne.* Epitaphs are meant to sum up the essence of the person and the life. Most of the things we worry about and lament daily have little or nothing to do with the overall value and meaning of our lives.

I think it can be helpful to consider what you would ultimately like your epitaph to be. I don't mean to sound depressing. Believe it or not, I'm really talking about living, not dying. I am asking you to examine how you are living today, in the here and now. You have the ability and privilege to write the many remaining chapters of your life that your epitaph will describe. While your life will certainly include unexpected events, you can decide how you will react to them.

■ Anne

Anne, a thirty-five-year-old acne sufferer, described how she had been slowly sucked into what she called the quicksand of life. A bad marriage, broken friendships, family betrayal, and a dead-end job all had taken their toll on her. Each of Anne's days began with bitterness and fatigue. She would go through the motions of her day anxious to return to the miserable but safe cocoon of her isolation.

All this changed abruptly at her office Christmas party. Anne agreed to go to the party only because she knew from previous years that anyone who missed the party was considered a loser. As a party joke, each staff member was assigned the task of anonymously creating a personality description of a coworker. They were printed on formal name tags and placed on a table near the entrance to the party. Each person was required to wear his or her badge prominently displayed for the duration of the party.

Anne looked somewhat anxiously for her name tag. She had been asked to suggest a name tag for her coworker Nancy. With little thought, she had jotted down "perky." What would hers be, she wondered? Ugly, pimply, pathetic? Finding her name tag, she quickly grabbed it, hoping no one else had seen it. Just as Anne was about to thrust it into her bag, Nancy took her arm and asked, "So, what does yours say?"

Anne stood rigidly, mortified at the prospect of having to show her name tag. Should she run, refuse, or simply surrender? Slowly, she held up the name tag and began to cry. There it was, printed in tasteful italics: "Stuck-up—too good for anybody." How could that be? It was just the opposite!

Walking as fast as she could, Anne struggled to hold back her tears as she made her way to the door. Finally, she found the exit. The brisk, cold air stung her cheeks as the tears flowed more freely. Leaning against the wall of the building, she felt limp. Suddenly, she stiffened as she felt a hand squeeze her arm. A soft, gentle, deep voice simply said, "Hey stuck-up, why the tears?" It was Frank, a longtime coworker with whom she had shared little conversation over the years. She knew him only as a nice, quiet guy.

Anne struggled to pull herself together and regain her controlled and aloof posture. A sea of emotions flooded her consciousness. She wanted so badly to run and hide, but at the same time, she was so hungry for companionship and acceptance. She looked at Frank and said, "I'm not stuck-up, and I'm not too good for anybody. I am just so scared of being hurt and feel so unattractive. I seem to be living in a cocoon, removed from all the happiness in life. I am so angry at what I have become. Please forgive me. I'm sorry."

As Anne turned to walk away, this near total stranger took both of her hands and said, "You know what comes from cocoons? Beautiful butterflies. Maybe it's your turn." Frank, apparently an angel of mercy, began to tell Anne his own tale of woe. He had been married for ten years— happily married, he thought. Returning from work early one day, he found his wife and his best friend in a devastatingly compromising position. A year of emotional pain and torment culminated in a divorce. The last five years had been, for Frank, a near mirror image of Anne's life.

Few words were spoken after Frank completed his story. They embraced and held one another for a very long time. Years of pain, fear, and anger had left them both so starved for closeness and warmth. Finally, their tight embrace slowly loosened, and Frank looked at Anne's face. Suddenly remembering her acne, Anne turned away, and new tears emerged. Frank pulled her closer and asked if he had offended her. Anne pointed to her face and said, "These pimples are so hideous." Frank looked into her eyes and said, "I don't care. They are not who you are."

So, did they live happily ever after? Yep, they did. An idyllic life filled only with smiles, kindness, and steamy romance? Nope, not at all. They lived a great life with all the fighting, good and bad days, great and mediocre sex, and the occasional "What did I get myself into?" that all good relationships have.

The point of Anne's story is not that fairy-tale endings inevitably occur, nor that they are necessary to attain happiness. The real point is that accepting yourself as a work in progress and living life in spite of your perceived imperfections is a necessary ingredient for a full and meaningful life. Anne's story could have ended just as happily had she made a new platonic friendship or become an active member in a work, school, social, or religious group. Any of those endings would provide human contact, sharing, warmth, laughter, and new experiences.

Anne had escaped her largely self-imposed cocoon and begun the process of living her life and, in so doing, rewriting her epitaph. No longer would "Stuck-up—too good for anybody" be the way in which those who knew her viewed her. Instead, more likely it would read "Embraced her life and those around her with warmth and passion."

Now it is your turn. Choose to live your life to the fullest each and every day. If your yesterdays have been filled with stress and sadness, begin to make small, incremental, positive changes that will improve your tomorrows.

Resources

ACNE INFORMATION

DermNet
A good Web site with information about all types of acne.
www.dermnet.org.nz

SkinCarePhysicians.com
A good Web site for information about common dermatologic
conditions.
www.skincarephysicians.com

The American Academy of Dermatology
Offers the latest research.
www.aad.org

ACNE SUPPORT

Acne Support Group
www.m2w3.com/acne

ACNE SELF-HELP STRESS MANAGEMENT

Acne Self-Help CD
A relaxation and guided imagery exercise developed and narrated by the author. Available at www.yardleyderm.com.

ROSACEA INFORMATION

Brownstein, Arlen, and Donna Shoemaker. 2001. *Rosacea: Your Self-Help Guide.* Oakland, Calif.: New Harbinger Publications.

National Rosacea Society
www.rosacea.org

GENERAL STRESS MANAGEMENT

Kabat-Zinn, Jon. 2002. *Mindfulness Meditation: Cultivating the Wisdom of Your Body and Mind.* New York: Simon & Schuster Audio.

Biofeedback Certification Institute of America
A good source for information about biofeedback. Can help you locate a certified biofeedback therapist.
www.bcia.org

The Mind Body Medical Institute
Herbert Benson's Mind Body Medical Institute; provides information about mindfulness meditation and home programs.
www.mbmi.org

Yoga Directory
Useful for locating yoga centers.
www.yogadirectory.com/Centers_and_Organizations

References

Adebamowo, C. A., D. Spiegelman, F. W. Danby, A. L. Frazier, W. C. Willett, and M. D. Holmes. 2005. High school dietary intake and teenage acne. *Journal of the American Academy of Dermatology* 52(2):207–14.

American Academy of Dermatology. 2005. Acne. http://www.aad.org/ NR/rdonlyres/19AB2C1C-B726-4BC9-8E7A-3C1CBDF79CFA/0/ Acne.pdf.

Basset, I. B., D. L. Pannowitz, and R. S. Barnetson. 1990. A comparative study of tea tree oil versus benzoyl peroxide in the treatment of acne. *Medical Journal of Australia* 153:455.

Baumann, L. 2001. Cosmeceutical critique: Soy and its isoflavones. *Skin and Allergy News* 32(8):17.

Benson, H. 2000. *The Relaxation Response: Updated and Expanded* (Twenty-fifth Anniversary Edition). New York: HarperCollins.

Boone, L. C., and G. E. Pierard. 1998. Digital image analysis of the effect of topically applied linoleic acid on acne microcomedones. *Clinical and Experimental Dermatology* 23(2):56–58.

Chiu, A., and A. B. Kimball. 2003. The response of skin disease to stress: Changes in the severity of acne vulgaris as affected by examination stress. *Archives of Dermatology* 139(7):897–900.

Cowley, G. 2002. The science of happiness. *Newsweek*, September 16, 46–48.

Cunliffe, W. J. 1986. Acne and unemployment. *British Journal of Dermatology* 115:379–83.

Draelos, Z. D. 2005. *Topical photoprotection.* Presented at the annual meeting of the American Academy of Dermatology. New Orleans, Louisiana.

Dunlop, K. J., and R. S. Barnetson. 1995. A comparative study of isolutrol versus benzoyl peroxide in the treatment of acne. *Australian Journal of Dermatology* 36(1):13–15.

Fried, R. G., and T. F. Cash. 1998. Cutaneous and psychological benefits of alpha hydroxy acid use. *Perceptual and Motor Skills* 86:137–38.

Gold, M. 2005. *Acne treatment with photodynamic therapy.* Presented at the annual meeting of the American Academy of Dermatology. New Orleans, Louisiana.

Gollnick, H., W. Cunliffe, D. Berson, B. Dreno, A. Finlay, J. J. Leyden, A. R. Shalita, and D. M. Thiboutot. 2003. Management of acne: A report from a global alliance to improve outcomes in acne. *Journal of the American Academy of Dermatology* 49(1):S1–S2.

Goulden, V., G. I. Stables, and W. J. Cunliffe. 1999. Prevalence of facial acne in adults. *Journal of the American Academy of Dermatology* 41:577–80.

Gupta, M. A., and A. K. Gupta. 1998. Depression and suicidal ideation in dermatology patients with acne, alopecia areata, atopic dermatitis, and psoriasis. *British Journal of Dermatology* 139:846–50.

———. 2001a. Dissatisfaction with skin appearance among patients with eating disorders and nonclinical controls. *British Journal of Dermatology* 145(1):110–13.

———. 2001b. The psychological comorbidity in acne. *Clinics in Dermatology* 19:360–63.

Harper, J. C., and D. M. Thiboutot. 2003. Pathogenesis of acne: Recent research advances. *Advances in Dermatology* 19:1–10.

Jick, S., H. M. Kremers, and C. Vasilakis-Scaramozza. 2000. Isotretinoin use and risk of depression, psychotic symptoms, suicide, and attempted suicide. *Archives of Dermatology* 136:1231–36.

Jowett, S., and T. Ryan. 1985. Skin disease and handicap: An analysis of skin conditions. *Social Science Medicine* 20:425–29.

Kellett, S. C., and D. J. Gawkrodger. 1999. The psychological and emotional impact of acne and the effect of treatment with isotretinoin. *British Journal of Dermatology* 140:273–82.

Lasek, R. J., and M. M. Chren. 1998. Acne vulgaris and the quality of life of adult dermatology patients. *Archives of Dermatology* 134:454–58.

Layton, A. M., C. A. Henderson, and W. J. Cunliffe. 1994. A clinical evaluation of acne scarring and its incidence. Abstract. *Clinical and Experimental Dermatology* 19:303–8.

Leung, L. H. 1995. Pantothenic acid deficiency as the pathogenesis of acne vulgaris. *Medical Hypotheses* 44(6):490–92.

Liu, J-C., M. Seiberg, J. Miller, J. J. Wu, S. Shapiro, and R. Grossman. 2001. Applications of soy in skin care. In *Proceedings of the Tenth EADV Congress, Munich.* Skillman, N.J.: Johnson & Johnson Consumer Products Worldwide.

Logan, A. C. 2003. Omega-3 fatty acids and acne. *Archives of Dermatology* 139(7):141–42.

Motley, R. J., and A. Y. Finlay. 1989. How much disability is caused by acne? *Clinical and Experimental Dermatology* 14:194–98.

Physicians' Desk Reference. 2005. Montvale, N.J.: Thomson Healthcare.

Plewig, G., and A. M. Kligman. 2000. *Acne and Rosacea.* 3rd ed. New York: Springer-Verlag.

Rapp, D. A., G. A. Brenes, and S. R. Feldman. 2004. Anger and acne: Implications for quality of life, patient satisfaction, and clinical care. *British Journal of Dermatology* 151:183–89.

Robertson, R. G., and M. Montagnini. 2004. Geriatric failure to thrive. *American Family Physician* 70:343–50.

Rubinow, D. R. 1987. Reduced anxiety and depression in cystic acne patients after successful treatment with oral isotretinoin. *Journal of the American Academy of Dermatology* 17:25–32.

Sadock, B. J., and V. A. Sadock. 2001. *Kaplan and Sadock's Pocket Book of Clinical Psychiatry*. 3rd ed. Philadelphia: Lippincott, Williams, and Wilkins.

Snider, B. L., and D. F. Dieteman. 1974. Pyridoxine therapy for premenstrual acne flare. *Archives of Dermatology* 110(1):130–31.

Spitz, R. A. 1945. Hospitalism. In *The Psychoanalytic Study of the Child*, Vol. 1, edited by R. S. Eissler. New York: International Universities Press.

Sulzberger, M. B., and S. H. Zaidens. 1948. Psychogenic factors in dermatologic disorders. *Medical Clinics of North America* 32:669–73.

Syed, T., and A. Q. Zulfiqar. 2001. *Treatment of acne vulgaris with 2 percent polyphenone (epigallocatechin gallate or green tea extract) in cream*. Poster at the annual meeting of the American Academy of Dermatology. Washington, D.C.

Taylor, S. 2005. Hormal management of acne. Data presented at the annual meeting of the American Academy of Dermatology. New Orleans, Louisiana.

Trattner, E. 2002. Alternative medicine. In *Cosmetic Dermatology: Principles and Practice*, edited by L. Baumann and E. Weisberg. New York: McGraw-Hill.

Wong, R. C., S. Kang, and J. L. Heezen. 1984. Oral ibuprofen and tetracycline for the treatment of acne vulgaris. *Journal of the American Academy of Dermatology* 11(6):1076–81.

Zouboulis, C. C., and M. Bohm. 2004. Neuroendocrine regulation of sebocytes: A pathogenetic link between stress and acne. *Experimental Dermatology* 13 suppl. 4:31–35.

Some Other
New Harbinger Titles

The Cyclothymia Workbook, Item 383X, $18.95

The Matrix Repatterning Program for Pain Relief, Item 3910, $18.95

Transforming Stress, Item 397X, $10.95

Eating Mindfully, Item 3503, $13.95

Living with RSDS, Item 3554 $16.95

The Ten Hidden Barriers to Weight Loss, Item 3244 $11.95

The Sjogren's Syndrome Survival Guide, Item 3562 $15.95

Stop Feeling Tired, Item 3139 $14.95

Responsible Drinking, Item 2949 $18.95

The Mitral Valve Prolapse/Dysautonomia Survival Guide,
Item 3031 $14.95

Stop Worrying Abour Your Health, Item 285X $14.95

The Vulvodynia Survival Guide, Item 2914 $15.95

The Multifidus Back Pain Solution, Item 2787 $12.95

Move Your Body, Tone Your Mood, Item 2752 $17.95

The Chronic Illness Workbook, Item 2647 $16.95

Coping with Crohn's Disease, Item 2655 $15.95

The Woman's Book of Sleep, Item 2493 $14.95

The Trigger Point Therapy Workbook, Item 2507 $19.95

Fibromyalgia and Chronic Myofascial Pain Syndrome, second edition,
Item 2388 $19.95

Kill the Craving, Item 237X $18.95

Rosacea, Item 2248 $13.95

Thinking Pregnant, Item 2302 $13.95

Call **toll free, 1-800-748-6273,** or log on to our online bookstore at **www.newharbinger.com** to order. Have your Visa or Mastercard number ready. Or send a check for the titles you want to New Harbinger Publications, Inc., 5674 Shattuck Ave., Oakland, CA 94609. Include $4.50 for the first book and 75¢ for each additional book, to cover shipping and handling. (California residents please include appropriate sales tax.) Allow two to five weeks for delivery.

Prices subject to change without notice.